Quantum Integrative Medicine for Brain Injury

A Clinician's Guide

Dr. Sarah Young
IMD, DHS, PhD, MS, CCC-SLP

Table of Contents

Dr. Sarah Young, IMD, DHS, PhD, MS, CCC-SLP

How to Use This Guide

This manual includes color-coded callout boxes throughout each chapter to support quick reference and clinical clarity. Each box highlights a key insight, action, or reflection to help you confidently apply integrative concepts in practice.

> **Action Step.** A specific clinical or implementation action to apply immediately.
>
> **Clinician Tip.** A best-practice insight, practical shortcut, or professional suggestion.
>
> **Research Insight.** Key evidence, citations, or emerging science for unfamiliar or complex topics.
>
> **Teach-Back Tool.** A prompt clinicians can use to check patient understanding or engagement.
>
> **Mind-Body Reflection.** A reflective prompt for clinicians to support emotional intelligence, sensitivity, or embodiment in practice.
>
> **Caution.** A warning about clinical care risks, sensitivities, or contraindications.

A note on how to read the evidence in this book: throughout these chapters you will see claims labeled by the strength and population of their supporting evidence, distinguishing what has direct acquired-brain-injury (ABI) trial support from what is drawn from adjacent populations (stroke, healthy volunteers), from mechanistic or animal work, or from clinical reasoning and original synthesis. Where a tool is promising but not yet established for ABI specifically, it is labeled investigational rather than presented as settled. This labeling is deliberate. It lets you weigh each recommendation for your own setting rather than accepting or dismissing the integrative model wholesale.

Introduction & Overview

Quantum Integrative Medicine for Brain Injury: A Clinician's Guide is the practical evolution of my dissertation, *Brain Injury: A Quantum Integrative Medicine Approach*. This guide transforms foundational academic research into an actionable resource for clinicians working with acquired brain injury (ABI). Combining evidence-informed science, clinical wisdom, and personal insight from my own journey and my patients' stories, it offers a tangible pathway for clinicians to bring Quantum Integrative Medicine (QIM) principles directly into practice.

Each chapter integrates clinical protocols, step-by-step intervention strategies, and illustrative case material, making abstract concepts relatable and applicable to everyday clinical scenarios. The case material in this book is presented as fictional educational composites drawn from commonly encountered clinical patterns, not as records of specific patients. This book moves beyond traditional symptom management, offering clinicians a comprehensive framework that addresses the full spectrum of ABI recovery: physical, emotional, cognitive, energetic, and relational.

QIM vs. Traditional Approaches

For those new to Quantum Integrative Medicine, it helps to understand how this approach expands upon traditional rehabilitation rather than replacing it. Conventional ABI treatment typically focuses on immediate symptom management: stabilizing acute injuries, reducing intracranial pressure, and mitigating functional deficits. These steps are essential. Contemporary practice increasingly recognizes, alongside them, the value of a broader approach that also attends to biological, psychological, social, and self-regulatory dimensions of recovery.

Quantum Integrative Medicine builds upon conventional neurorehabilitation by integrating:

- **Neurological repair.** Combining standard therapies (physical therapy, cognitive rehabilitation) with neuroplasticity-informed techniques.
- **Metabolic and nutritional support.** Addressing gut-brain disturbances, nutritional imbalances, and systemic inflammation common after ABI.
- **Bioenergetics and frequency therapies.** Using energy-based tools such as neurofeedback, low-level laser (photobiomodulation), and pulsed electromagnetic fields, with each labeled by its current evidence strength for ABI rather than presented uniformly.

- **Mind-body and consciousness-based approaches.** Engaging cognitive and emotional states through mindfulness, meditation, guided imagery, and expectation/placebo effects that have measurable physiological correlates.

Rather than replacing conventional medical care, QIM is intended to work alongside it, treating recovery as a multidimensional process that involves the whole neurophysiological and emotional life of the patient.

What This Guide Provides

This guide is structured for clinical application. It includes treatment approaches, structured assessment pathways, and practical strategies for incorporating QIM into daily patient care. Each chapter builds sequentially, from foundational frameworks and scientific principles toward explicit guidance on assessment and treatment.

Practical tools include:

- A working explanation of the **Five Bodies of Healing** (Physical, Vital, Mental, Supramental, Bliss) as a lens for whole-person assessment.
- Guidance for developing care plans informed by the **Five Pillars of Health** (Elimination, Assimilation, Immunity, Oxidation, Regeneration).
- A structured **"Day in the Life"** protocol that gives a tangible example of an integrative ABI routine, from morning hydration and mindfulness through daytime active regulation and therapy work to evening wind-down.

This practical orientation is meant to help clinicians translate theory into individualized, integrative care plans.

> **Caution: Misinterpreting Neuroplasticity.** Neuroplasticity is not inherently positive. Without guided structure, the brain can reinforce maladaptive pathways, and repetition of dysfunctional patterns can become entrenched. Support clients with intentional retraining and regular clinical feedback, not repetition alone.

Addressing Skepticism: Evidence and Clarity

Quantum Integrative Medicine draws on neuroscience, functional medicine, and bioenergetic tools to support brain-injury recovery. Because some of these approaches sit outside conventional rehabilitation, it is worth being direct about what the evidence does and does not show. The honest position is not that every QIM tool is proven for ABI, nor that integrative approaches are unfounded, but that the strength of evidence varies by tool and population, and each should be weighed on its own merits.

> **Research Insight.** The term "biofield" refers to the endogenous electromagnetic fields associated with living systems. This concept is used in integrative medicine as an organizing frame for energy-based interventions. It should be understood as a conceptual and hypothesis-generating framework rather than a fully established clinical mechanism; the strength of evidence differs sharply between measurable modalities (for example, EEG-based neurofeedback and PEMF) and more speculative interpretations. *(Evidence label: the biofield construct is hypothesis-level, an organizing frame rather than an established clinical mechanism.)*

A few clarifications for clinicians new to the language:

- **Biofield and electromagnetic signaling.** Just as EEG measures the electrical activity of the brain, some energy-based therapies (for example, PEMF) aim to influence cellular and neural function through electromagnetic stimulation. The measurable, device-based end of this spectrum has a real evidence base; the more speculative "subtle energy" end does not, and this book keeps the two distinct.
- **Quantum language, used carefully.** Terms borrowed from physics (entanglement, coherence) are used in integrative medicine largely as *metaphor* for mind-body interconnection and the influence of psychological state on physiology. They are not a claim that macroscopic quantum entanglement drives healing. Where this book uses such language, it does so as a conceptual lens, and the underlying clinical point (that emotional and cognitive states measurably affect physiology) stands on conventional psychophysiology, not on quantum mechanics.

Key supporting areas (with honest evidence labels)

- **PEMF therapy.** Studied for effects on neuroinflammation and recovery; evidence for ABI specifically is emerging rather than definitive, and is developed with population labels in Chapters 3, 4, and 8.
- **Neurofeedback.** EEG-based neurofeedback has a substantial literature for cognitive and emotional regulation; its ABI-specific evidence and its distinction from *diagnostic* qEEG are handled carefully in Chapters 2, 4, and 9.
- **Gut-brain interventions.** The gut-brain axis is well established as biology; evidence that microbiome-directed treatment improves ABI recovery *specifically* is not yet established, and is labeled as such in Chapter 6.

Common clinician concerns, answered directly

- *"QIM isn't scientifically validated."* Some component therapies (PEMF, neurofeedback, targeted nutrition, mindfulness-based neuroplasticity training) have meaningful peer-reviewed support; others are investigational. This book labels each rather than defending or dismissing the whole. The validity question is answered tool by tool, not as a package.
- *"Biofield therapies lack measurable outcomes."* Device-based modalities such as PEMF and neurofeedback do produce measurable biomarker and EEG changes; the strength and ABI-specificity of those outcomes vary and are labeled accordingly.
- *"Quantum concepts aren't clinically relevant."* The clinically relevant claim is the well-supported one: emotional state, expectation, and stress regulation measurably affect physiology and outcomes. That claim does not require quantum mechanics to hold, and this book does not rest it there.

The aim of this guide is to let clinicians apply integrative principles with clear eyes, knowing which tools are established, which are promising, and which remain investigational.

Chapter 1: Foundations of Quantum Integrative Medicine (QIM)

For decades, the treatment of acquired brain injury (ABI) was guided by a reductionist model: one that isolated symptoms, categorized impairments, and targeted specific deficits for management. This framework provided valuable tools for acute stabilization and functional retraining, especially in early recovery. Patients often leave these programs walking again, speaking more fluently, or regaining some independence. But many are still left with invisible wounds: lingering fatigue, emotional dysregulation, brain fog, or a profound disconnection from their pre-injury sense of self. Conventional rehabilitation, while necessary, often falls short of the full complexity of what it means to heal after a brain injury. It emphasizes mechanical repair over whole-person restoration, and can miss the interplay between mind, body, physiology, and the person's felt experience.

This is where Quantum Integrative Medicine (QIM) reframes the conversation. QIM views the brain not as a machine needing repair, but as part of a deeply interconnected system shaped by biological processes, physiological regulation, emotional states, and belief. Healing, in this model, is not merely about rewiring neurons. It is about restoring coherence across systems: neurologically, metabolically, emotionally, and in the person's sense of self and relationships. In QIM, factors such as trauma, social connection, purpose, and conscious engagement are not peripheral; they are central to recovery. Neurorehabilitation is not only clinical. It is human.

A note on the word "quantum." This book uses it the way integrative medicine generally does, as a frame for interconnection and for the measurable influence of mental and emotional states on physiology, rather than as a claim that macroscopic quantum mechanics governs healing. Where quantum language appears, read it as a conceptual lens. The clinical claims underneath it rest on conventional neuroscience, psychophysiology, and functional medicine, and are labeled by their evidence throughout.

> **Research Insight.** Neuroplasticity remains active well into adulthood, enabling the brain to reorganize following injury, particularly when therapy incorporates multisensory and cognitive engagement. *(Evidence label: experience-dependent plasticity is a well-supported principle. Popular texts on the subject are useful patient and clinician reading rather than primary evidence.)*

Historically, ABI recovery has operated under a "fix what's broken" philosophy: stabilize vitals, minimize physical disability, and teach compensatory strategies. These interventions are essential, but they often stop short of addressing why so many survivors feel "recovered but not restored." They meet functional milestones yet continue to experience loss of clarity, chronic fatigue, or mood disturbance that goes unaccounted for. Emerging work in neuroplasticity, the gut-brain axis, autonomic regulation, and mind-body medicine is expanding this view. The brain is not a fixed organ; it is highly plastic, capable of reorganizing in response to internal and external input. And healing is not strictly linear. It occurs across multiple layers of experience, from the physical to the emotional to the self-regulatory.

Recovery from brain injury takes more than physical therapy or medication. It takes a whole-body, whole-person approach, and that is what QIM is built to provide. Rather than focusing on one part of recovery in isolation, QIM attends to how systems in the body and brain interact, combining modern neurorehabilitation with established mind-body practice and carefully-labeled emerging therapies. For example, QIM draws on action-observation and motor-imagery approaches, dual-task exercises, and guided imagery to engage neuroplastic mechanisms; it addresses inflammation and oxidative stress by supporting the gut-brain axis, nutrition, and mitochondrial health; and it uses tools such as PEMF, neurofeedback, and photobiomodulation to support nervous-system regulation, each at its own level of evidence. Because emotion and mindset matter, QIM also includes mindfulness, breathwork, and visualization to support emotional regulation and expectation effects. None of this replaces conventional care. It works alongside it.

At the heart of QIM lies a claim with real support behind it: the therapeutic relationship is itself part of the treatment. The clinician's presence, empathy, and communication style can support or hinder recovery. Research in relationship-centered care indicates that when patients feel seen, heard, and included in their own care, they are more likely to engage, stay motivated, and follow through, with downstream effects on outcomes. Conventional models have often been top-down: clinicians prescribe, patients comply. But ABI survivors are not only managing cognitive deficits. They are often grieving a changed identity, living with invisible symptoms, and navigating profound emotional change. Rehabilitation that does not acknowledge these dimensions falls short.

The shift toward relationship-centered care recognizes that recovery is collaborative. Patients are active agents in their healing, not passive recipients. This means involving them in decisions, listening to their concerns, and adapting communication to their cognitive needs, moving from "this is what you need to do" toward "here are your options; what feels most supportive to you?" For patients with ABI, communication must be adaptive: clear, structured, and multimodal. Visual aids, step-by-step instructions, and teach-back methods support comprehension and retention when memory and processing speed are affected. Health literacy is not just a clinical task; it is relational. How we teach matters as much as what we teach.

1.1 The Whole-System View: What ABI Actually Disrupts

Acquired brain injury is more than a structural trauma. It is a multisystem disruption that affects the brain's metabolism, immune regulation, redox balance, gut-brain communication, and capacity for plasticity. Recovery depends on more than task repetition or time; it requires system-level support that addresses the biological breakdowns beneath the symptoms. Each of these threads gets its own chapter later in the book. This section is the map for finding them.

- **Metabolic dysfunction** is a hallmark of ABI. Impaired glucose uptake, mitochondrial fatigue, and reduced ATP production are associated with mental fog, energy crashes, and poor neural signaling (Prins & Matsumoto, 2014; Giza & Hovda, 2014). *(Developed in Chapters 5 and 6.)*
- **Neuroinflammation**, driven by chronically activated microglia, is associated with cognitive and emotional symptoms long after the initial trauma. Microglial responses after TBI are complex rather than uniformly harmful (Loane & Kumar, 2016). No single inflammatory marker identifies the cause of an individual patient's persistent symptoms; this is a population-level pattern, not an individual diagnostic tool. *(Developed in Chapter 3.)*
- **Oxidative stress** damages neurons through unchecked reactive oxygen species and lipid peroxidation, worsening fatigue and impairing learning (Hall et al., 2010). *(Developed in Chapter 3.)*
- **Gut-brain axis disruption** is often overlooked. Dysbiosis, intestinal permeability, and vagal dysfunction are associated with altered serotonin regulation, nutrient absorption, and immune balance (Carabotti et al., 2015; Cryan et al., 2019). These are general reviews of gut-brain biology, not evidence that microbiome-directed treatment improves ABI recovery specifically. *(Developed in Chapter 6.)*
- **Neuroplasticity** is the cornerstone of recovery, but plasticity is experience-dependent, and maladaptive pathways can form without proper stimulation (Kolb & Gibb, 2011, a developmental-neuroscience review, cited for its general experience-dependent-plasticity principles rather than as ABI-specific evidence). The nervous system learns through more than physical execution: observation, imagery, and modeled behavior recruit overlapping elements of the brain's action-perception and

motor-planning networks (Rizzolatti & Craighero, 2004), a foundation this book returns to in its approach to sequencing intervention. *(Developed in Chapter 9.)*

1.2 A Multidimensional Model: The Five Realms

The multisystem disruption above (metabolic, immune, oxidative, gut-brain, and neuroplastic) is the biological layer of a larger pattern. Human beings are multidimensional, and healing that addresses only the physical misses most of what recovery actually requires. The **Five Realms** framework organizes that larger pattern and serves as the overarching map for this entire book. Ordered from the most subtle to the most dense, the Realms are:

1. **Essence** - the deepest layer of identity, meaning, and coherence; the felt sense of being oneself.
2. **Awareness** - conscious cognition, belief, attention, and perception.
3. **Field** - the relational and energetic surround: connection, environment, and the person's regulatory relationship with the world around them.
4. **Flow** - autonomic and energetic regulation; the movement of state and energy through the nervous system.
5. **Form** - the physical body and its physiological processes.

The Five Realms are not a competing model to the frameworks that follow. They are the container. Two more specific and long-standing frameworks nest inside them, each doing a distinct job: the **Five Bodies of Healing**, which describe *what is happening* across the subtle-to-dense span of a person, and the **Five Pillars of Health**, which describe the *physiological functions* operating within Form. The Five Bodies map onto the Realms directly; the Five Pillars live entirely within Form. Both are developed in full below as standalone frameworks, because each is clinically usable on its own, and each earns its place in the model.

The practical payoff of the Realms is immediate. A symptom or an intervention does not have only one location. It has a Realm of origin, and within Form specifically, a functional Pillar it works through. That is the multidimensional argument made concrete rather than asserted. It is the frame the rest of this book uses when a chapter's content clearly belongs to one Realm (Chapter 4's autonomic work lives in Flow; Chapter 3's neuroinflammation and Chapter 6's mitochondrial work live in Form) and when it deliberately crosses Realms (Chapter 7's trauma work bridges Flow and Field; Chapter 10's identity work is centered in Essence and Awareness but shaped by everything beneath it).

1.3 The Five Bodies of Healing

In conventional medicine, healing is often compartmentalized. We are trained to separate mind from body, to treat symptoms in isolation, and to measure success by physical milestones. In ABI recovery, this fragmented approach frequently falls short. Healing does not occur in a vacuum, and it does not only move from the body upward. Recovery can also begin from the top down. Beliefs, emotions, relationships, and regulatory states actively shape biology. What happens in awareness has tangible effects on what happens in neurons.

This is the core idea behind the Five Bodies of Healing. Rooted in older healing systems and increasingly informed by modern neuroscience, this model invites us to view patients as more than physical beings. ABI is not just a disruption of neurons or motor function. It affects energy and autonomic flow, emotional regulation, cognition, and the core of a person's identity. To facilitate true, lasting recovery, we work across all of these dimensions.

The principle of downward causation helps explain why. In contrast to a strict "body-first" model, where physical healing is expected to lead to cognitive and emotional improvement, downward causation holds that higher-order experiences, belief, purpose, emotional repair, can drive biological change. Recovery is dynamic and systems-driven, not merely mechanical. The Five Bodies, from subtle to dense, are the Bliss Body, the Supramental Body, the Mental Body, the Vital Body, and the Physical Body. Mapped onto the Realms: Bliss and Supramental sit within Essence and Awareness, Mental within Awareness, Vital within Flow, and Physical within Form.

The Bliss Body. This is the deepest layer of consciousness: the space of meaning, emotional integration, and sense of purpose. After ABI, many individuals feel unmoored, questioning their identity or place in the world, disconnected not only from others but from themselves. Patients who find meaning in recovery, through spirituality, community, mindfulness, or personal growth, often show greater resilience and engagement. Practices like meditation, gratitude, and social bonding can reduce stress-driven physiological load and support the states associated with adaptation and healing. Cultivating inner steadiness or purpose does more than lift mood; it has physiological correlates.

> **Research Insight.** Finding meaning in recovery, through spirituality, mindfulness, community, or personal growth, is associated with better emotional resilience and cognitive engagement. Contemplative practice supports self-regulation, and gratitude, loving-kindness, and social connection are associated with neurochemical and physiological changes that favor recovery. *(Evidence label: these associations come from contemplative-neuroscience and affective-science research, not from ABI-specific outcome trials.)*

The Supramental Body. This layer governs higher cognition, intuition, and belief. It is where the recovery mindset takes root. What a patient expects about recovery can shape physiological reality. Placebo research shows that expectation alone can modulate pain perception and neurotransmitter activity and can influence functional outcomes. Visualization, in which patients mentally rehearse speech, movement, or a task, engages overlapping neural networks to those used in physical execution. Cognitive reframing helps shift self-defeating thoughts into workable narratives, lowering fear-based inhibition. When patients believe recovery is possible, and are actively supported in that belief, they are more able to engage the work that makes it possible.

> **Research Insight.** Expectation functions as a physiological variable, not only a psychological one. Placebo-neuroscience research shows positive expectation can modulate brain activity, reduce pain perception, and engage endogenous opioid and dopamine systems. Motor imagery and mental rehearsal activate motor-planning networks overlapping with actual performance. Cognitive reframing is associated with reduced limbic reactivity and improved executive regulation. *(Evidence label: well supported in general populations; the magnitude of effect in ABI specifically varies.)*

The Mental Body. This reflects cognition, perception, and emotional regulation, domains often significantly disrupted by ABI. Survivors may struggle with anxiety, irritability, or low mood, both because of what has happened and because ABI can alter emotional-processing networks. Mindfulness-based cognitive therapy and neurofeedback are useful here; they can support attentional stability and emotional balance. Emotional dysregulation is not a peripheral concern. It directly affects sleep, autonomic function, and the conditions for plasticity. Healing the Mental Body is therefore part of functional recovery, not separate from it.

> **Research Insight.** The Mental Body, cognition, perception, and emotional regulation, is among the most affected domains after ABI, reflecting changes in circuits governing attention, mood, and executive function. Emotional dysregulation is linked to limbic and prefrontal alterations. Interventions such as MBCT and neurofeedback are associated with reduced rumination and improved emotional self-regulation. *(Evidence label: supported in general and adjacent clinical populations; ABI-specific outcome data are more limited.)*

The Vital Body. Here we enter autonomic regulation and the flow of state and energy, governed largely by the autonomic nervous system. ABI often dysregulates this domain, producing chronic fatigue, poor stress tolerance, and dizziness, signs of an overwhelmed or poorly regulated ANS. The Vital Body can be retrained. Heart-rate-variability (HRV) biofeedback supports vagal tone and helps rebalance sympathetic and parasympathetic activity; breathwork and somatic practices reduce hyperreactivity and support oxygen delivery; PEMF is sometimes used here to support cellular energy, at its own evidence level. Without stabilizing this layer, patients frequently plateau in other therapies. The nervous system must feel safe before the brain can reorganize. This is the clinical heart of Chapter 4.

> **Research Insight.** The Vital Body includes the autonomic and energetic systems governing physiological balance, often disrupted after ABI. HRV biofeedback is associated with enhanced vagal tone and emotional regulation; somatic practices such as diaphragmatic breathing lower physiological stress load. PEMF is associated with effects on mitochondrial function and inflammation, at an emerging evidence level for ABI. *(Evidence label: HRV biofeedback and breath-based regulation have reasonable general support; the PEMF claims here sit at an emerging level for ABI.)*

The Physical Body. The most visible and traditionally emphasized domain, and the seat of conventional rehabilitation: motor retraining, cognitive and speech-language therapy, anti-inflammatory nutrition, and conditioning. These tools are critical, and they work best when they are not working alone. Patients who have also addressed the higher bodies, aligning belief, emotional regulation, and autonomic stability, often respond more readily to physical interventions, because their nervous systems are more prepared for change. Aligning the higher bodies helps unlock the full value of physical rehabilitation.

Many ABI survivors report feeling fragmented, as though mind and body are no longer in sync. This is more than metaphor; it is a lived experience with correlates in connectivity and regulation. Applying the Five Bodies lets clinicians build personalized, multidimensional plans that integrate the whole person, pairing neurological repair with meaning-making, breathwork, and visualization alongside functional therapy. We begin to see not a patient with symptoms, but a person navigating a healing process. The Five Bodies framework is not a rejection of conventional rehabilitation. It is the connective structure that lets us engage the whole reality of brain injury and recovery.

1.4 The Five Pillars of Health

Healing from ABI is not a straight, linear process. It is more like traveling a five-lane highway, with each lane a physiological system that must function well to support the journey. These five systems, Elimination, Assimilation, Immunity, Oxidation, and Regeneration, form the Five Pillars of Health. They provide the internal scaffolding that allows neuroplasticity to take hold, cognition to recover, and the body to rebalance. If even one pillar is weak or dysregulated, recovery can be delayed or incomplete. Working together, they create the conditions for durable healing. Within the Five Realms, all five Pillars live inside Form: they are the functional processes of the physical layer.

Most conventional programs focus almost entirely on functional recovery, helping patients walk, talk, remember, and complete daily tasks. Those goals are critical, but they overlook a key truth: however advanced the therapy, it will not hold if the body's internal terrain is inflamed, nutrient-deprived, or metabolically imbalanced. The Five Pillars stabilize that foundation so other therapies can be more effective.

> **Research Insight.** The Five Pillars of Health, Assimilation, Elimination, Regeneration, Oxidation, and Immunity, are a foundational framework in integrative and functional medicine. In ABI recovery, disruptions such as impaired detoxification, malabsorption, oxidative stress, or chronic inflammation can slow progress, and support for microbiome health, mitochondrial function, and immune modulation can help restore the physiological balance that enables neuroplastic change. *(Framework attribution: the Pillars are widely used in functional medicine; the ABI-specific application is the author's clinical synthesis.)*

Elimination is the body's ability to clear what no longer serves it: metabolic waste, neurotoxic byproducts, environmental exposures, and inflammatory debris, which can accumulate after injury and hinder repair. The brain's glymphatic system clears waste primarily during deep sleep, and ABI often impairs it, contributing to fog and fatigue. Supporting elimination is practical: optimize sleep, maintain hydration, encourage lymphatic flow through gentle movement, and support digestive regularity, since the gut and brain communicate closely via the vagus nerve.

> **Research Insight.** Circadian rhythms regulate hormonal cycles, sleep architecture, and synaptic remodeling, all relevant to recovery. Circadian disruption is associated with increased neuroinflammation and impaired memory consolidation. Interventions such as morning light exposure, time-restricted eating, and structured sleep hygiene help restore circadian alignment. *(Evidence label: the circadian and neuroinflammation link rests substantially on animal-model work; the interventions themselves are low-risk and widely endorsed.)*

Assimilation is absorbing and using the nutrients the recovering brain needs. Neurorehabilitation is energy-intensive; every synaptic change depends on a steady supply of substrate. Yet ABI often disrupts digestion, absorption, and blood-sugar stability. Replenishing brain-relevant nutrients (omega-3s, magnesium, B vitamins, polyphenols), supporting gut repair, and stabilizing blood sugar with balanced meals all support this pillar.

Immunity is about regulating inflammation. Inflammation is part of healing, but chronic neuroinflammation is a major obstacle to recovery, impairing cognition, disrupting sleep, and slowing plasticity. Management is multifaceted: an anti-inflammatory, polyphenol-rich diet; targeted compounds such as curcumin and resveratrol to modulate microglial activity; vagal support; and, importantly, stress regulation through breathwork, mindfulness, and HRV work to shift the body out of a sympathetic-dominant state that sustains inflammatory cascades.

Oxidation centers on mitochondrial health, the energy-producing engines of the cell. The brain consumes roughly 20% of the body's energy while accounting for about 2% of its weight, and after ABI mitochondrial function is often impaired, contributing to fatigue, slowed cognition, and emotional instability. Nutritional support (CoQ10, NAD+ precursors, alpha-lipoic acid), oxygen-supporting practices (breathwork, red-light therapy, and, at an investigational level for chronic mild TBI, HBOT), and circadian alignment can support mitochondrial output.

Regeneration is the activation of neuroplasticity itself: the body's capacity to rebuild and rewire. Plasticity is not passive; it must be sparked and guided, and it thrives only when conditions are right. Neuroplasticity-driven therapies (dual-task training, cognitive retraining, coordinated movement), neuromodulation (neurofeedback, entrainment, PEMF at their own evidence levels), and, critically, deep sleep, when the brain consolidates memory and performs cellular repair, all belong to this pillar. Without adequate quality sleep, plasticity stalls, which is why sleep optimization is non-negotiable here.

Together, the Five Pillars are the physiological foundation of ABI recovery. Where conventional therapy asks whether function is improving, QIM also asks whether the body is prepared for healing, whether the systems that support plasticity are actually in place. When elimination works, the brain clears waste; when assimilation is optimized, nutrients reach cells; when immunity is regulated, inflammation stops sabotaging progress; when oxidation is supported, energy is available for repair; and when regeneration is activated, the brain changes in lasting ways. The stronger this foundation, the better the results other therapies can produce.

> **Mind-Body Reflection: Beliefs About Healing.** Ask: "Where do my beliefs about healing come from, and how have they changed?" Invite clients to reflect too. Change often begins with a shift in perception.

1.5 Relationship-Centered Care and Health Literacy

Healing from a brain injury is never only a medical process. It is a human one, unfolding in relationship with clinicians, caregivers, and the self, and the quality of those relationships can support or hinder recovery. Conventional models have focused on treating symptoms, helping patients walk, speak, or remember, but ABI recovery is about rebuilding a life: identity, emotion, trust, belonging. A person may regain language and still feel invisible; walk independently and still feel ungrounded. The emotional and psychological impact of brain injury is profound and often under-addressed. Relationship-centered care moves beyond symptom management toward whole-person healing, placing human connection at the center of the encounter.

In practice, this means recognizing the individual behind the diagnosis. It begins with listening, not only to medical detail but to the patient's story: what they are struggling with emotionally, how the injury has affected their sense of self, what recovery means to them. It involves shared decision-making, inviting patients into planning rather than handing down protocols, asking "what feels manageable for you right now?" For survivors who have lost a sense of autonomy, regaining even small control can be transformative.

One of the most overlooked barriers in ABI rehabilitation is health literacy. This is not just whether a patient can read a handout; it is whether they can understand, remember, and apply what is communicated. Brain injury often affects memory, attention, processing speed, and executive function. Patients may nod during an appointment and forget everything by the time they leave, or feel overwhelmed by jargon and multi-step instructions. This reflects the neurological reality of ABI, not intelligence or motivation. When clinicians do not adapt, patients disengage.

> **Clinician Tip: Use Metaphors.** Use patient-friendly metaphors for neurological processes. Neuroplasticity, for example, can be compared to "rewiring a garden path," fostering understanding without oversimplifying the science.

Supporting health literacy starts with clear, plain language and the translation of medical concepts into everyday terms. Visual tools (diagrams, illustrated checklists, written summaries) bridge comprehension gaps. The teach-back method, inviting patients to explain instructions in their own words, confirms understanding and strengthens retention. Involving caregivers matters, since they often bridge clinic instructions and real-world follow-through. When information is delivered in accessible, cognitively friendly ways, patients can take a more active role, and that sense of agency often supports engagement.

Beyond communication lies empathy. Expertise is vital but not sufficient. Healing requires trust, and trust is built through emotional presence. For many survivors, life has been upended; they are grieving both what they have lost and what remains uncertain. Being heard without interruption offers relief. Statements like "I hear you, and I can imagine how frustrating this is" do more than feel good: they support physiological safety, lowering stress and increasing readiness to engage. Emotional safety lets the nervous system move out of survival mode into a state where the work of recovery is possible.

Trust also means adapting to the invisible challenges ABI creates. Rather than labeling difficulty with decision-making, emotional regulation, or planning as resistance, relationship-centered clinicians meet patients where they are, adjusting communication and offering choices. The shift from "you have to do this" to "which of these options feels right to you?" is small but meaningful. It supports autonomy and motivation.

> **Clinician Tip: Make Goals Functional and Relatable.** Use real-world language to co-create goals. Instead of "improve verbal expression," try "ask for help at the store" or "tell my daughter a story." Functional phrasing supports motivation, retention, and daily carryover.
>
> **Caution: One-Size-Fits-All Protocols.** Be cautious with rigid or prepackaged protocols. Integrative care must respond to each client's biology, history, and lived experience. Individualization is essential to avoid harm or stagnation.

1.6 Supporting Skill Mastery in ABI Recovery

Healing after brain injury involves more than regaining lost function; it means relearning how to learn. Many patients must start over with daily tasks, memory strategies, emotional regulation, or speech and movement. Understanding how people progress through skill development lets clinicians tailor interventions, reduce frustration, and protect emotional safety during a vulnerable process.

One practical model is the Conscious Competence framework, which describes four stages:

6. **Unconscious incompetence.** The patient does not yet know what they do not know. This can present as reduced awareness, common in ABI due to anosognosia; patients may believe they are functioning normally while struggling with attention, memory, or regulation.
7. **Conscious incompetence.** Insight emerges. Recognizing deficits can bring grief, anger, or discouragement. This is a critical window for motivational interviewing, compassionate coaching, and trauma-informed care.
8. **Conscious competence.** Skill development begins. Patients can complete tasks but must concentrate to succeed, like someone using a memory notebook who still needs reminders and feedback.
9. **Unconscious competence.** The skill is internalized. This is the goal, though not every patient reaches it with every skill, and clinicians should continue to encourage autonomy and celebrate incremental gains.

Most survivors move between these stages across different domains at once. A patient may reach unconscious competence with a pill organizer while remaining at conscious incompetence with impulse control. Recognizing this variation prevents unrealistic expectations and supports goal-based rehabilitation. To support skill mastery: use visual and tactile cues to reinforce routines; offer structured repetition with built-in feedback; validate emotional responses to setbacks; and empower patients to track their own gains through journaling, apps, or video. Recovery is not about perfection but about progress that feels possible.

> **Research Insight: Seeing Is Firing.** Action observation engages the action-perception system and can facilitate motor-relevant cortical activity even without overt movement, a principle behind action-observation therapy, mirror therapy, and virtual-reality rehabilitation. The magnitude and durability of clinical benefit vary by application and population, and are developed with evidence labels in Chapters 4 and 9. *(Evidence label: the mirror mechanism is well characterized as neuroscience (Rizzolatti & Craighero, 2004); it is a conceptual basis for these therapies rather than ABI outcome evidence in itself.)*

1.7 Learner Types and Representation Styles

Not every patient processes information the same way, and after ABI this variability is more pronounced. Challenges in attention, memory, and executive function often interfere with learning through standard methods, so clinicians must deliver information intentionally, adapting to each patient's cognitive and sensory processing. Understanding learner types does more than aid communication; it can be the difference between a disengaged patient and one who feels empowered.

One widely used model, VARK, classifies learners as visual, auditory, reading/writing, and kinesthetic. Visual learners benefit from charts, diagrams, and color-coding; auditory learners from spoken explanation, rhythm, and dialogue; reading/writing learners from written materials and structured notes; kinesthetic learners from tactile or movement-based strategies such as gesture and hands-on activity. Many survivors benefit from a blended, multimodal approach, especially when one channel has been compromised. A patient with working-memory difficulty may benefit from hearing instructions while viewing a printed aid; a kinesthetic learner with attentional challenges may improve comprehension by physically engaging, tapping fingers to count syllables or tracing letters while rehearsing. (VARK describes preferences and is best used as a flexible clinical tool rather than a fixed rule; the value here is the deliberate use of multisensory delivery, which has a stronger evidence base than strict learning-style matching.)

Representation systems go beyond preference; they reflect how the injured brain encodes, processes, and retrieves information. After ABI, a patient may no longer learn as they once did, so clinicians observe closely and stay flexible, asking "how do you best remember things now?" or "would it help to draw this out together?" Honoring each patient's learning style is a form of respect and a tool for change, building self-efficacy and supporting the neural reorganization that recovery depends on.

> **Clinician Tip.** For patients with memory impairment, combine visual and kinesthetic input, for example tapping a finger for each word repeated aloud, or "drawing" a concept on the tabletop. These cross-body techniques support multisensory integration and can improve attention, encoding, and working memory.
>
> **Caution: Trauma Activation.** Mind-body practices, reflection prompts, and even breathwork can surface unresolved trauma. Ensure clients have grounding tools, informed consent, and access to psychological support. Know when to pause or refer to trauma-trained clinicians.

1.8 Neuroplasticity and Consciousness-Based Healing

For a long time, recovery from ABI was seen as fixed: once the damage was done, patients were thought to hit a ceiling. Research over recent decades has overturned that belief, largely because of one quality of the brain: neuroplasticity, its ability to adapt, reorganize, and form new pathways based on experience. This is an ongoing process, not a one-time event. Healing from ABI is less about returning to who someone was than about building a workable new version of themselves, one connection at a time. And consciousness, thoughts, beliefs, and focus, actively shapes that process. Repeated signals forge pathways, so what we think, feel, and attend to influences the structure and function of the brain. This is the foundation of consciousness-based healing.

The brain does not sharply distinguish a vividly imagined experience from a real one at the level of motor planning. Visualizing picking up a cup or crossing a room engages circuits overlapping with actually doing it, a phenomenon known as motor imagery. This connects to the action-observation system, engaged when we watch others perform an action we want to relearn, which is the basis of action-observation therapy and mirror therapy, useful in hemiparesis and aphasia. Consciousness-based healing goes beyond movement: guided imagery, mindfulness, and the expectation of improvement engage reward systems, and belief is therefore not only hopeful thinking but has neurochemical correlates. The brain needs more than time to engage plasticity; it needs intentional, meaningful repetition. The more consciously a patient engages, through visualization, mindful practice, and emotional regulation, the more robust the changes tend to be.

Action Step: Tools that help engage neuroplasticity.

- **Mental rehearsal.** Visualizing movement or speech engages motor and language circuits, helping bridge intention and action.
- **Mindfulness meditation.** Supports attention and executive function while calming stress reactivity.
- **The placebo effect, reframed.** Not tricking the brain, but harnessing expectation: when patients anticipate improvement, reward and endogenous-opioid systems can support engagement.
- **Gratitude and positive expectation.** Associated with an emotional environment that favors learning and adaptation.

When patients actively participate, practicing focused mental exercises, training attention, working with emotion, their brains become more responsive and ready to change. There is a neurochemical foundation here: dopamine supports motivation and learning (and can be encouraged by celebrating small wins or gamified rehab); serotonin supports emotional stability (supported by mindfulness, breathwork, and nutrition); acetylcholine supports attention and learning (stimulated by challenging cognitive and motor tasks); and glutamate supports memory encoding (engaged through aerobic exercise and skill repetition). All are influenced by lifestyle and internal state. Even a few minutes of deep breathing at the start of a session can lower stress load and prime the brain for learning. One of the most practical principles in rehabilitation is Hebb's insight that neurons that fire together wire together: the more we practice, especially with full focus, the stronger the pattern. And "practice" is not only physical movement; watching, imagining, and affirming supportive beliefs engage the brain similarly, which is why guided visualization, self-talk, and reframing sit alongside conventional exercises.

Clinician Tip: Symptom Assessment Across the Five Bodies. Invite patients to score each Body (Physical, Vital, Mental, Supramental, Bliss) on a 1-10 scale weekly. This helps identify patterns across domains and lets clients track subtle shifts in their trajectory.

Self-awareness matters throughout. After ABI, people often feel disconnected from themselves and may struggle to recognize progress, but journaling, guided reflection, and clinician feedback can rebuild insight. This is about more than regaining function; it is about reconnecting to a sense of self. Neuroplasticity is not just a clinical term. It is an invitation for patients to become co-creators in their healing, and a reminder for clinicians to see each patient as a whole person capable of meaningful change.

1.9 Energy Medicine and Frequency-Based Tools

We have long understood the body through a biochemical lens, but that is only part of the story. The body is also bioelectrical: cells maintain electrochemical gradients, neurons signal electrically, and the brain operates on frequency-specific wave patterns. Given this, therapies that engage the body's electrical and regulatory systems can plausibly play a role in recovery, particularly after ABI. In the QIM model, "energy medicine" spans a wide range of tools, and it is essential to be honest that they do not share one evidence level. The device-based, measurable end of this spectrum (for example, EEG-based neurofeedback and PEMF) has a real and growing literature; the more speculative "subtle energy" end does not, and this book keeps the two clearly distinct rather than presenting them as equivalent.

> **Research Insight (framing).** The "biofield" is used in integrative medicine as an organizing concept for endogenous electromagnetic activity and energy-based interventions. It is best treated as a conceptual and hypothesis-generating frame, not an established clinical mechanism. When patients describe fatigue, fog, or feeling "off" despite normal scans, those experiences are real and worth addressing; attributing them specifically to "biofield dysregulation" is interpretation, and the interventions below are recommended on their own measurable merits rather than on that interpretation. *(Evidence label: biofield and primo-vascular claims in this area are hypothesis-level or contested rather than established anatomy or mechanism.)*

Pulsed electromagnetic field (PEMF) therapy delivers low-frequency pulses to brain and body and has been studied for effects on mitochondrial function, inflammation, blood flow, and neuronal repair. After ABI the brain often enters a relative energy crisis, with reduced ATP and increased oxidative stress, and PEMF is proposed to support recovery in this context. Early work in stroke and TBI populations is promising for cognition and emotional regulation, but the ABI-specific evidence is emerging rather than definitive, and PEMF should be offered as a supportive, still-developing tool.

Neurofeedback lets patients observe brainwave activity and learn to modulate it. ABI can disrupt normal rhythms, and neurofeedback aims to train the brain toward more regulated patterns, for example supporting calmer states in post-injury anxiety. It has a substantial general literature; its ABI-specific evidence is developed, with the important distinction between diagnostic qEEG and neurofeedback as intervention, in Chapters 2 and 9.

Brainwave entrainment uses sound or light to guide the brain toward target frequencies. Tools such as binaural beats or rhythmic light may support relaxation, attention, mood, and sleep with little active effort, and are non-invasive and generally well tolerated. **Vibration and sound-based tools**, tuning forks, vibroacoustic therapy, and infrared/red-light therapy, are used to support parasympathetic balance and tissue-level repair; red-light therapy (photobiomodulation) has the more developed evidence base of this group, while others are more preliminary. **Sound practices** such as humming and chanting can stimulate vagal activity and support regulation, with downstream effects consistent with the vagus nerve's role in brain-body communication.

Energy medicine is a synergistic partner to conventional care, not a substitute for it. A session might open with a few minutes of PEMF to support nervous-system readiness, followed by breathwork to settle stress, then neurofeedback and dual-task training, closing with entrainment or vibroacoustic support for integration. Layer by layer, the treatment activates, regulates, and restores, while keeping each tool at its honest level of evidence. Widening the clinical lens to include the bioelectrical side of healing opens possibilities for supporting mood, cognition, and nervous-system regulation, and for engaging patients as active participants, provided we remain clear about what is established, what is promising, and what remains investigational.

> **Research Insight.** Multimodal care that integrates metabolic, cognitive, and regulatory therapies is associated with improvements in attention, emotional regulation, and sleep quality, outcomes central to ABI recovery. *(Evidence label: this association rests on clinical observation and adjacent literatures rather than controlled ABI trials of multimodal programs.)*

Chapter 1 Quick-Reference Guide and Summary

Core concepts.

- **Quantum Integrative Medicine (QIM).** Combines conventional neurorehabilitation with whole-person, multidimensional approaches, including neurometabolic support, frequency-based tools, and consciousness-based practice, each held to its own evidence level.
- **The Five Realms** (Essence, Awareness, Field, Flow, Form) provide the overarching map, from subtle to dense.
- **The Five Bodies of Healing** (Bliss, Supramental, Mental, Vital, Physical) describe healing across those Realms.
- **The Five Pillars of Health** (Elimination, Assimilation, Immunity, Oxidation, Regeneration) are the physiological functions within Form that support plasticity and recovery.

- **Relationship-centered care** prioritizes empathy, empowerment, health literacy, and collaboration.
- **Neuroplasticity and consciousness-based healing** use mental rehearsal, mindfulness, and visualization to actively engage plastic change.
- **Energy medicine and frequency-based tools** (PEMF, neurofeedback, entrainment, photobiomodulation) support regulation and coherence, distinguishing measurable modalities from speculative ones.

> **Action Step.** As you move into clinical application, choose one new concept or technique to explore at a time, integrating it slowly, observing, reflecting, and adjusting. Sustainable transformation happens through small, intentional shifts.
>
> **Action Step.**
>
> - Blend dual-task cognitive and motor activities into daily rehabilitation to support global network activation and real-world plasticity.
> - Use visual supports and teach-back to reinforce understanding, reduce cognitive overload, and improve adherence.
> - Integrate mindfulness-based practices (breathwork, guided imagery, movement-based meditation) to support emotional regulation and cognitive clarity, helping clients find regulation strategies that feel safe.
> - Explore environmental regulation and grounding (time in nature, earthing, reasonable EMF hygiene) as accessible supports, while trained clinicians may add neurofeedback or PEMF.
> - Introduce the Five Bodies as an educational tool for patient insight and engagement, creating a multidimensional map that extends beyond symptom tracking into empowered participation.

Chapter 2: Understanding Acquired Brain Injury (ABI)

Concept map for this chapter. Chapter 2 is deliberately more concise than the original, because several of its topics are developed at full length elsewhere rather than twice. Nothing was dropped; everything relocated is mapped here so you do not have to hunt for it.

Original Chapter 2 topic	Where it is developed in full
Evolution of ABI rehabilitation	**Here**, §2.1
Observer effect and clinician presence	**Here**, §2.2; relational application in Ch.10
Metabolic dysfunction and the brain's energy crisis	Summarized here §2.3; full treatment in **Ch.3 §3.3** (Metabolism domain) and **Ch.7 §7.9** (mitochondrial support)
Neuroinflammation	Summarized here §2.3; full treatment in **Ch.3 §3.3** and **Ch.7 §7.2**
Oxidative stress	Summarized here §2.3; full treatment in **Ch.3 §3.3**
Gut-brain axis, dysbiosis, permeability, vagal function	**Here**, §2.4 in full; protocols in **Ch.4 §4.4**; symptom management in **Ch.7 §7.10**
Neuroplasticity tools and neurotransmitter modulation	**Here**, §2.5; protocol detail in **Ch.4 §4.2**; sequencing in **Ch.9 §9.4**
PEMF, light, sound, neurofeedback	**Here**, §2.6 in full; clinical application in **Ch.4 §4.3**; emerging developments in **Ch.8**
Comparative models of rehabilitation	**Here**, §2.7 in full

The rule applied: each topic is developed in full in exactly one place and summarized where it first becomes relevant, so a reader following the book in order encounters the idea when they need it and the detail when they can use it.

2.1 From Mechanism to Meaning: The Evolution of ABI Rehabilitation

Acquired brain injury has undergone a profound reclassification in the past decade. Once viewed primarily as an acute medical event, defined by visible trauma, immediate neurological deficits, and short-term stabilization, it is now increasingly understood as a chronic, lifelong condition. Survivors often face ongoing cognitive, emotional, metabolic, and autonomic challenges that extend far beyond the injury itself. This shift has changed not only how outcomes are measured but how care must be delivered.

Historically, ABI rehabilitation followed a mechanistic model rooted in biomedicine. Protocols emphasized symptom control, structural stabilization, and isolated retraining of function. The brain was treated like a machine: if a part failed, the goal was to bypass it or recruit adjacent areas. This approach offered clear benefits in acute care, saving lives, restoring motor function, and addressing gross deficits, but it fell short in addressing the invisible, lingering impacts of brain injury: brain fog, chronic fatigue, mood instability, relational disconnection, and loss of identity.

In the 1980s and 1990s, the emergence of neuropsychology and person-centered care marked the beginning of a shift. Clinicians began to acknowledge that rehabilitation concerned more than muscles and memory scores; it concerned the person's lived experience. Cognitive rehabilitation expanded to include attention, executive function, and psychosocial adaptation, and emotional support, therapeutic alliance, and quality of life entered the conversation. Even these expanded frameworks, though, often focused on symptom management rather than systems-level healing.

The past two decades have brought another transformation, toward integrative, systems-based, and consciousness-informed approaches. With the growth of functional medicine, trauma-informed care, and neuroplasticity research, it has become clear that recovery is neither linear nor isolated to any one system. ABI affects, and is affected by, everything from gut health and inflammation to relationship dynamics, emotional regulation, and belief. The brain does not heal in a vacuum. It heals within a matrix of physiology, psychology, environment, and awareness.

Quantum Integrative Medicine emerges as the next step in this evolution, not as a replacement for existing models but as a synthesis drawing from neuroscience, energy-based tools, trauma-informed psychology, and older wisdom traditions. It works across levels, from neurotransmitters and mitochondria to self-efficacy and coherence, on the premise that to restore the brain we must also support the person.

2.2 The Observer Effect: Your Role in Recovery

Quantum physics introduced a striking idea: observation can influence what is measured. This principle, the observer effect, describes how particles behave differently under measurement. In healthcare, the observer effect functions as a powerful **metaphor** for how clinician presence, attention, and intention shape the healing encounter.

> **Evidence label.** This section uses quantum language deliberately as analogy. The clinical claims below do not depend on literal quantum mechanics operating at the scale of clinical care; they rest on relational neuroscience, psychophysiology, and placebo/expectancy

> research, which are well established in their own right. Sources in this area are hypothesis-level or contested rather than established mechanism, and this book does not rely on them. The author's synthesis, that the clinician is inside the system rather than outside it, is preserved as original clinical reasoning.

In QIM, the therapeutic relationship is not merely a backdrop for treatment; it is an active field in which healing unfolds. When a clinician enters a session with focused attention, curiosity, and compassion, the patient's nervous system often begins to regulate more efficiently. Neuroception, the nervous system's subconscious appraisal of safety, responds to cues of attunement and emotional presence. That perception of safety supports parasympathetic activity, which in turn favors the physiological conditions for repair and plastic adaptation. The clinician's role as observer is not passive. It creates a relational field that influences outcomes in real time.

Quantum entanglement adds a second layer, again as model rather than mechanism. Entanglement describes linked particles whose states correspond regardless of distance. In QIM, it offers a metaphor for the interconnection between clinician and patient, body and mind, thought and biology. We do not claim brain-injury recovery hinges on literal particle entanglement. The instructive parallel is simply this: healing happens in relationship. When clinicians and patients engage in shared intention, believing in recovery, visualizing progress, co-creating goals, they participate in a system that affects biological expression.

This framework also helps explain the measurable effects of placebo, expectancy, and intention-setting in ABI rehabilitation. Patients' belief in recovery correlates with improved functional outcomes, and when clinicians express confidence in a patient's capacity to heal, patients often perform better across treatment modalities. These outcomes are not merely psychological; they involve neurotransmitter, immune-signaling, and network-level changes. The brain responds not only to therapy but to meaning, belief, and relational context.

The observer effect may partly shape neuroplasticity itself. Mental imagery, visualization, and mindfulness engage cortical circuits without physical movement. When a patient visualizes walking, motor planning regions activate. Observation, attention, and relational attunement are not extras; they are part of how the brain changes.

> **Research Insight.** Relational neuroscience and polyvagal-informed work support the view that attuned clinician attention influences the patient's autonomic state, supporting calm, connection, and the physiological conditions for repair. Placebo and expectancy research demonstrates that shared clinician-patient expectation of progress is associated with improved outcomes across diverse modalities, reflecting real changes in neurotransmitters,

> inflammatory markers, and plasticity. *(Evidence label: placebo and expectancy effects are well established across modalities. Polyvagal theory is a widely used clinical framework whose specific evolutionary claims remain debated; its clinical utility for framing safety and regulation is what is used here.)*

2.3 Neuropathophysiology of ABI: Key Mechanisms of Dysfunction

ABI does not disrupt the brain in a single moment; it initiates a cascade that continues long after the acute event. Traditional models focus on visible impairments like motor loss or speech difficulty, but many of the most persistent symptoms, fatigue, brain fog, chronic pain, mood instability, and cognitive sluggishness, are not merely structural. They reflect an internal environment thrown off balance by metabolic disruption, chronic inflammation, and oxidative stress.

In most rehabilitation settings, therapy centers on rebuilding skills. Those goals matter, but they do not explain why some patients plateau or remain stuck in cycles of exhaustion. Without addressing the internal mechanisms below, even excellent therapy protocols can feel like pushing uphill against biology.

> **Clinician Tip: Teaching the Five Pillars.** Turn each of the Five Pillars into a self-assessment discussion. Ask: "Which pillar feels strongest for you right now? Which feels least supported?" Use the answers to set priorities in care.

Metabolic dysfunction: the brain's energy crisis. The brain is the body's most energy-demanding organ, requiring constant oxygen, glucose, and mitochondrial support. After injury this system falters. Glucose metabolism slows, contributing to mental fatigue, poor concentration, and reduced processing speed, while mitochondrial function declines and ATP becomes harder to produce. The brain's ability to use alternative fuels such as ketones is often compromised as well. This explains why so many survivors describe overwhelming fatigue or thinking "through molasses." It is not a motivation problem; it is underpowered neurons. Restoring energy metabolism is therefore foundational. Ketogenic approaches are proposed to provide alternative fuel; mitochondrial cofactors such as CoQ10, NAD+ precursors, and alpha-lipoic acid are used to support cellular energy; and oxygen-supporting therapies (breathwork, red-light therapy, and HBOT at an investigational level) are used to support bioenergetics. *(Evidence label: the metabolic cascade after TBI is well characterized (Giza & Hovda, 2014; Prins & Matsumoto, 2014). The specific interventions above range from reasonable-mechanistic to investigational for ABI; ketogenic and mitochondrial-cofactor strategies in ABI rest largely on mechanistic and preclinical work rather than* *definitive human ABI trials. The originally cited Poff et al. source could not be verified and has been removed as a citation; the underlying claim is retained here as hypothesis-level.)*

Neuroinflammation: the persistent fire. Inflammation is part of healing, but after ABI it often becomes stuck in the "on" position. Microglia mobilize to clear damage but remain activated rather than resolving, producing a smoldering chronic inflammation that continues to disrupt function. This affects multiple domains: cognition, memory, and processing speed; neurotransmitter balance, contributing to emotional volatility, anxiety, and depression; and autonomic function, contributing to poor heart-rate variability, temperature sensitivity, and unexplained fatigue. As inflammation lingers it feeds oxidative stress and mitochondrial dysfunction. Interventions target the root: omega-3s, curcumin, and resveratrol to modulate microglial activity and pro-inflammatory cytokines, and vagal support, HRV training, and mindfulness-based stress reduction to shift the nervous system toward a more restorative state. *(Evidence label: microglial responses after TBI are complex rather than uniformly harmful (Loane & Kumar, 2016); no single inflammatory marker diagnoses an individual patient's symptoms. Curcumin's poor natural bioavailability means formulation matters clinically. Chapter 3 develops this in full.)*

> **Research Insight: A Note on Oxalates.** Oxalate is naturally present in many plant foods (spinach, almonds, beets). Dietary oxalate warrants clinical attention in people with hyperoxaluria, recurrent calcium-oxalate kidney stones, or specific metabolic disorders. A proposed role in ABI-related neuroinflammation and mitochondrial stress remains **hypothesis-level and unestablished for this population**, and low-oxalate dietary approaches should not be presented to ABI patients as an evidence-based recovery intervention. This material is retained rather than removed, with its speculative status stated plainly. *(Evidence label: the supporting literature comes from non-ABI populations and does not establish this approach for brain injury.)*

Oxidative stress: the silent neurotoxin. Oxidative stress works like rust in the nervous system, a slow breakdown driven by reactive oxygen species the body cannot clear quickly. After ABI, antioxidant defenses are often compromised. Because the brain consumes more oxygen than any other organ and is rich in delicate unsaturated fats, it is especially vulnerable. When reserves such as glutathione, superoxide dismutase, and catalase are depleted, lipid peroxidation destabilizes membranes and disrupts synaptic signaling, contributing over time to memory difficulty, reduced learning capacity, and mental fatigue (Hall et al., 2010). Support includes alpha-lipoic acid, resveratrol, and glutathione-supporting strategies, alongside breathwork and red-light therapy to support oxygen metabolism. HBOT is sometimes considered here; its evidence in chronic mild TBI is investigational and mixed, and is examined in detail in Chapter 3.

Reframing recovery: from deficit to dysfunction to healing. What we see in clinic, slurred speech, emotional lability, memory lapses, is the tip of the iceberg. Beneath it lies metabolic exhaustion, immune overdrive, and oxidative stress, the hidden terrain that so often explains stalled recovery. When patients plateau it is rarely for lack of effort. Pushing harder with conventional therapy will not break the cycle unless core systems are supported. A systems-based view uses nutrition to stabilize blood sugar and fuel availability, mitochondrial support to rebuild the energy grid, HRV training and vagal support to regulate inflammation, antioxidants to protect neurons, and patient education so people understand why these layers matter. When patients understand their internal terrain, they participate with new clarity and motivation.

2.4 The Gut-Brain Axis, Intestinal Permeability, and Vagal Function

The brain and gut are connected through a bidirectional network known as the gut-brain axis. The great majority of the body's serotonin is produced in the gut, and the gut microbiome participates in neurotransmitter synthesis, immune function, and inflammatory regulation.

After ABI, this axis is often disrupted. Injury can shift microbiome composition (dysbiosis), increase intestinal permeability, and impair vagal function. These changes are associated with persistent neuroinflammation, cognitive difficulty, emotional volatility, and fatigue.

Dysbiosis. After injury, beneficial populations such as *Lactobacillus* and *Bifidobacterium* often decline while less favorable organisms expand. This shift is associated with reduced availability of GABA, serotonin, and dopamine precursors and with increased lipopolysaccharide (LPS) production, an inflammatory signal that can contribute to neuroinflammatory responses.

Increased intestinal permeability. Often called leaky gut, this allows undigested particles, microbial products, and inflammatory agents into circulation, potentially aggravating already vulnerable neural tissue and impairing absorption of nutrients the brain needs for repair, including omega-3 fatty acids, amino acids, and B vitamins. Nutrients used to support barrier integrity include L-glutamine, colostrum, zinc carnosine, and polyphenol-rich foods.

Vagal dysfunction. The vagus nerve is the primary conduit between central and enteric nervous systems, modulating digestion, mood, and inflammation. After ABI it is often dysregulated, reducing parasympathetic tone, slowing motility, and favoring sympathetic dominance. Vagal support techniques, diaphragmatic breathing, humming, cold exposure, and HRV training, can help restore parasympathetic regulation.

> **Evidence label.** The gut-brain axis is well established as biology (Carabotti et al., 2015; Cryan et al., 2019, both general reviews). What is **not** established is that microbiome-directed treatment improves ABI recovery specifically; human ABI intervention data remain limited (see Pathare et al., 2020, which carries its own human-study limitations). "Leaky brain" and LPS-mediated neuroinflammation are mechanistically plausible and actively researched rather than clinically confirmed pathways in ABI. Recommend gut-supportive care as reasonable and low-risk, not as proven ABI treatment. Chapter 6 develops this fully.

2.5 Supporting Self-Healing with Neuroplasticity Tools

Neuroplasticity is the brain's capacity to adapt, rewire, and reorganize in response to experience. It is the mechanism by which recovery after ABI occurs. Without it, rehabilitation would be limited to compensation; with it, meaningful recovery becomes possible.

After injury the brain enters a period of both vulnerability and potential. Existing networks are disrupted, but the conditions for new circuits also open. Because plasticity is experience-dependent, the direction of change, adaptive or maladaptive, is shaped by daily habits, emotional states, therapeutic input, and belief. Time alone does not guarantee improvement; recovery depends on intentional stimulation that activates adaptive pathways.

Mental training and cognitive therapy. Structured cognitive challenge is among the most effective ways to guide plastic change. Dual-task training, performing simultaneous motor and cognitive tasks, mirrors real-world demand and engages integrative functions such as executive control and cognitive flexibility. Mental imagery and visualization offer additional tools, especially when physical limitation prevents full participation: imagining a movement engages motor-planning pathways overlapping with performing it, letting patients begin retraining before full function returns.

Neurotransmitter modulation. The success of plastic interventions is tied to the brain's neurochemical environment. Dopamine facilitates reward-based learning, goal-directed behavior, and attentional focus, supported by exercise and meaningful activity. Acetylcholine supports memory encoding and retrieval, supported by cognitive challenge and, in some protocols, citicoline or alpha-GPC. Serotonin supports emotional regulation, impulse control, and sleep, supported by mindfulness, natural light exposure, and adequate dietary tryptophan. *(Evidence label: these are general neuropharmacological principles. Note specifically that citicoline was tested directly in TBI in the COBRIT trial (Zafonte et al., 2012, n=1213) and did not show benefit; that negative result is retained deliberately. L-tyrosine and related catecholaminergic strategies remain plausible hypotheses without dedicated ABI trial support.)*

Self-directed techniques. Recovery does not stop when a session ends. Mindfulness-based cognitive therapy trains non-judgmental observation of thought and feeling, supporting emotional regulation and executive control. Mirror therapy uses visual feedback to engage motor pathways, and guided mental rehearsal helps consolidate patterns of successful speech, movement, or daily task performance. These practices turn passive recovery into an active process in which patients become partners.

> **Research Insight: The Glymphatic System.** During deep sleep, glymphatic clearance removes metabolic waste from neural tissue via cerebrospinal fluid flow. This system is most active during slow-wave sleep, tying sleep quality directly to brain clearance. Supporting glymphatic function through sleep optimization and hydration is a reasonable and low-risk part of recovery care. *(Evidence label: glymphatic biology is well established in animal models and increasingly in humans; specific ABI-recovery outcomes from "glymphatic-targeted" intervention are not established.)*
>
> **Teach-Back Tool.** "How would you describe neuroplasticity in your own words? Can you give an example of how practice might help the brain rewire?"

2.6 PEMF, Light, Sound, and Neurofeedback: What They Do

The brain functions through electrical rhythms that coordinate thought, movement, perception, and autonomic regulation. After ABI these patterns are often disrupted, contributing to cognitive fog, emotional instability, sleep disturbance, and dysautonomia. Frequency-based therapies aim to support healthier oscillatory activity and cellular function rather than targeting symptoms directly.

Brainwave entrainment and binaural beats. The brain operates across frequency bands associated with different states. Delta (0.5-4 Hz) is associated with deep sleep and restorative processes, often diminished in patients with insomnia or poor clearance. Theta (4-8 Hz) is associated with emotional processing, learning, and integration. Alpha (8-12 Hz) supports relaxed focus and mental clarity, and reduced alpha coherence is common after ABI. Beta (12-30 Hz) supports focused cognition and executive function, with too little contributing to sluggish thinking and excess high-beta associated with anxiety and irritability. Entrainment tools, binaural beats, isochronic tones, and neurofeedback, aim to support healthier oscillation. *(Evidence label: binaural beats and entrainment have modest, mixed evidence for relaxation and attention in general populations and little ABI-specific outcome data; they are low-risk adjuncts, not established ABI treatments.)*

Neurofeedback provides real-time feedback on brainwave activity, training the brain toward more regulated patterns. It has a substantial general literature for attention and emotional regulation (see Gruzelier, 2014). Two clinical cautions carry through the book: qEEG findings are not specific to TBI and should not independently establish diagnosis, determine severity, or prescribe a neurofeedback protocol; and diagnostic EEG/qEEG and neurofeedback as intervention are related but not interchangeable.

PEMF therapy delivers low-frequency electromagnetic pulses, proposed to support mitochondrial respiration and ATP production, modulate pro-inflammatory signaling and microglial overactivation, and support plasticity. Work in stroke and TBI populations reports improvements in cognitive endurance, fatigue, and autonomic regulation. *(Evidence label: emerging. Much of the supporting literature is mechanistic, preclinical, or from adjacent populations; ABI-specific controlled evidence remains limited.)*

Photobiomodulation (red and near-infrared light) targets mitochondrial cytochrome c oxidase, supporting ATP synthesis and oxygen utilization and reducing oxidative stress. Small studies report improvements in cognitive performance and mood in neurological conditions, including a frequently cited pair of chronic-TBI case reports (Naeser et al., 2011). *(Evidence label: promising, with the most developed mechanistic rationale of this group, but resting on case reports and small open-protocol studies rather than controlled trials; not an established standard.)*

Vibration and sound. Tuning forks, vibroacoustic therapy, and practices such as humming and chanting are used to support parasympathetic tone and regulation. These are low-risk comfort-and-regulation tools; their specific ABI-outcome evidence is minimal, and they should be offered as such.

> **Caution: Client Overexertion.** Clients with brain injury often push too hard too early, leading to overstimulation, fatigue crashes, or emotional regression. Monitor tolerance closely and build in structured rest to balance effort with recovery.

2.7 Comparing Traditional, Biopsychosocial, and QIM Models

Over the past century, ABI care has evolved through distinct models, each shaped by the prevailing medical philosophy of its time. Each contributed insight; none alone captures ABI as a multisystem, chronic condition.

The **Traditional model** emerged from the biomedical paradigm, focusing on acute stabilization, symptom suppression, and physical restoration. It excels in emergency response and structural intervention, saving lives, managing crises, restoring motor function, but tends to overlook the cognitive, emotional, and regulatory impairments that surface months or years later.

The **Biopsychosocial model** gained prominence in the late twentieth century, recognizing that biological mechanisms, psychological resilience, and social support all shape recovery. By integrating cognitive rehabilitation, mental health services, and social reintegration, it addressed many gaps in traditional care. It still tends to underweight autonomic and energetic regulation, trauma imprinting, and plastic potential as active drivers of recovery.

Quantum Integrative Medicine builds on both, adding frequency-based tools, neuroenergetics, consciousness-informed practice, and personalized systems biology. It treats recovery as a matter of both repairing tissue and reestablishing coherence across domains.

Focus	Model	Strengths	Limitations
Structural damage, symptom control	Traditional biomedical	Emergency stabilization, surgery, pharmacology	Reductionist; underaddresses emotional, cognitive, and regulatory dimensions
Biological, psychological, and social domains	Biopsychosocial	Includes mental health, family systems, cognitive therapy	Limited focus on neuroimmune, bioenergetic, and consciousness-informed drivers
Multisystem regulation, neuroplasticity, energy, and consciousness-based healing	Quantum Integrative Medicine (QIM)	Combines structural, functional, energetic, and meaning-based care; individualized	Requires clinician training across modalities; not yet mainstream; component evidence varies by tool

Clinically, QIM offers depth for survivors who remain symptomatic after standard rehabilitation. By integrating nervous-system regulation, nutritional neuroscience, frequency-based therapy, self-tracking tools, and patient empowerment, it aims to support function across all five Bodies. It does not ask clinicians to abandon conventional care; it invites them to expand the toolbox. In this light, QIM is not a rejection of ABI rehabilitation. It is its extension.

Chapter 2 Quick-Reference Guide and Summary

Core concepts.

- **Evolution of the field.** ABI is now understood as a chronic, multisystem condition rather than a discrete acute event.

- **The observer effect.** Clinician presence, attention, and expectation measurably shape the encounter and the patient's regulatory state. Used here as model and metaphor, resting on relational neuroscience and placebo/expectancy evidence.
- **Neuropathophysiology.** Metabolic disruption, neuroinflammation, and oxidative stress form the hidden terrain beneath persistent symptoms.
- **Gut-brain axis.** Dysbiosis, permeability, and vagal dysfunction are plausible amplifiers of persistent symptoms; supportive care is reasonable, not proven ABI treatment.
- **Neuroplasticity tools.** Dual-task training, mental imagery, mirror therapy, and neurochemical support, with citicoline's negative COBRIT result stated plainly.
- **Frequency-based tools.** PEMF, photobiomodulation, entrainment, and neurofeedback, each at its own evidence level, with qEEG/neurofeedback distinctions preserved.
- **Model comparison.** QIM as extension of, not replacement for, traditional and biopsychosocial care.

Practical clinical actions.

- Support neurotransmitter balance through individualized, clinician-supervised strategies rather than generic supplementation.
- Use empathy-driven communication and action-observation-informed activities to support social and emotional rehabilitation.
- Integrate patient-centered mental imagery and positive reinforcement to engage expectancy effects deliberately and ethically.
- Apply frequency-based treatments (PEMF, neurofeedback) individually and with appropriate training, remembering that qEEG does not by itself prescribe a protocol.
- Educate patients using simplified analogies, checking comprehension with teach-back rather than assuming it.

Chapter 3: The QIM Neurorehabilitation Model

Traditional rehabilitation often takes a bottom-up approach, prioritizing physical function first and addressing cognitive and emotional rehabilitation later. That model has merits, but it does not account for the interconnected nature of brain healing. Recovery is not linear, nor is it confined to isolated systems. The nervous system, metabolism, immune function, cognition, and a person's sense of self all interact, influencing the pace and depth of neurological repair.

The QIM Neurorehabilitation Model operates on the principle that healing happens at multiple levels simultaneously. It integrates metabolic restoration, neuroimmune balance, cognitive restructuring, relationship-centered care, and consciousness-informed practice into a single framework. It does not view the brain as a machine requiring rewiring; it treats the brain as a responsive, adaptive, interconnected system. Recovery involves more than retraining motor circuits; it means creating the conditions in which neuroplasticity, metabolic resilience, and regulatory stability can take hold.

Two models, two questions. This book contains two of the author's original translational frameworks, and they answer different questions. The **Five Core Domains** in this chapter describe **where** care is directed: which territory of the person a given intervention addresses. The **Three-Phase Model** in Chapter 9 (Priming, then Intensive Neural Activation, then Reinforcement) describes **how** care unfolds over time: the sequence in which those interventions are introduced. Neither supersedes the other. A clinician uses the Domains to decide what to address and the Phases to decide when. Both are presented as the author's clinical-organizing synthesis, an original translational contribution rather than a claim of independently validated protocol; individual components carry their own evidence labels.

3.1 The Three Operating Principles

Before the Domains themselves, three interdependent principles govern how the model is applied. They are not domains of intervention but the conditions under which intervention works.

Relationship-centered care. Recovery is relational as well as biological. The quality of the therapeutic alliance influences neurobiological outcomes: trust, empathy, and shared decision-making are associated with reduced stress load, better autonomic regulation, and greater engagement with treatment. A patient who feels emotionally safe is more able to participate fully and less likely to be operating from a state of threat. Trauma-informed care extends this by acknowledging the emotional and psychological impact of ABI, creating conditions in which self-directed neuroplasticity tools can actually be used. A brain in survival mode has limited capacity for the demanding work of recovery; safety and relational trust are prerequisites, not amenities.

Consciousness-based healing. The mind is an active participant in plastic change. Visualization, mindfulness, and expectation are not merely supportive practices. Mental rehearsal engages motor-planning pathways overlapping with physical movement even in the absence of mobility. Mindfulness practice supports emotional regulation and executive control. Patient belief influences motivation, engagement, and neurochemical state. The placebo effect, often dismissed, is a measurable phenomenon rooted in expectancy. When patients hold the possibility of recovery, they contribute to the conditions that support it. *(Evidence label: expectancy and motor-imagery effects are well supported in general populations; the author's synthesis, that consciousness is integral rather than incidental to biology, is original clinical reasoning presented as such.)*

Integrative neuroscience. Cognitive deficits, fatigue, and slowed processing are often surface expressions of deeper dysfunction: neuroimmune dysregulation, mitochondrial impairment, and disrupted signaling. Supporting the brain's energy systems, addressing chronic inflammation, and using frequency-based interventions can improve cellular function and network coherence. Interventions must also be personalized. Each brain heals differently, and an individualized, data-informed approach targets the patient's actual physiological profile rather than applying generic protocols.

> **Clinician Tip: Teamwide Symptom Check-ins.** Implement a weekly interdisciplinary check-in to discuss symptom changes and adapt protocols. Collaborative tracking ensures consistency, reveals patterns, and strengthens alignment across modalities and disciplines.

3.2 Domain One: Energy

The brain is more than a biochemical organ; it is an electrically active system. Neurons communicate through oscillating signals that shape cognition, motor coordination, mood, and perception. After ABI these rhythms are often disorganized, frequency patterns become unstable, and the brain struggles to maintain coherence across networks. This dysregulation contributes to lingering cognitive fatigue, emotional instability, and autonomic dysfunction.

Neuroelectric stimulation offers a direct route to modulating neural activity. ABI often produces either cortical hypoactivity (underactive, poorly integrated regions) or compensatory hyperactivity contributing to anxiety, insomnia, and poor focus. Transcranial direct current stimulation (tDCS) applies a low current to targeted regions and has been studied for effects on working memory and executive function. Transcranial magnetic stimulation (TMS) uses magnetic fields to modulate cortical activity and has established use in depression with promising work in post-stroke motor recovery. Cranial electrotherapy stimulation (CES) is a non-invasive option studied for anxiety and cognitive fatigue. These are most effective when combined with active cognitive rehabilitation rather than used alone. *(Evidence label: tDCS and TMS have substantial general literatures with real ABI-specific limitations; TMS for depression is established, while ABI-specific cognitive protocols remain investigational.)*

Brainwave optimization. Efficient brain function requires regions to communicate in coherent patterns. After ABI this synchronization is often disrupted, contributing to slowed processing and difficulty with complex tasks. Entrainment techniques (binaural beats, isochronic tones) use rhythmic auditory or visual stimuli to guide oscillatory activity, and neurofeedback provides real-time feedback allowing patients to retrain rhythms deliberately. *(Evidence label: neurofeedback has meaningful general support (Gruzelier, 2014) with important methodological debates (Thibault et al., 2016); entrainment tools are low-risk with modest and mixed evidence.)*

PEMF and photobiomodulation. PEMF delivers low-frequency electromagnetic pulses studied for effects on calcium signaling, ATP synthesis, and gene expression associated with neural repair, with animal TBI models showing reduced microglial activation and improved sensorimotor outcomes. Photobiomodulation targets mitochondrial cytochrome c oxidase, supporting cerebral blood flow, reducing oxidative damage, and improving neuronal viability in animal and early human work. *(Evidence label: both are emerging. Much support is preclinical or from adjacent populations; ABI-specific controlled human evidence remains limited.)*

Biofield-based approaches. Sound therapy, vibroacoustic therapy, tuning-fork work, humming, and chanting are used to support parasympathetic tone and emotional equilibrium, with vagal stimulation the most plausible mechanism. Early studies of biofield therapies report reductions in anxiety and stress markers. *(Evidence label: these remain under-researched in neurology, with small studies and significant methodological limitations. They are reasonable low-risk comfort and regulation tools, not established ABI treatments, and this book does not present them as equivalent to the device-based modalities above. GDV and Bio-Well-type "biofield imaging" should not be presented to patients as validated diagnostic technology.)*

> **Teach-Back Tool.** "Imagine a friend asks what PEMF therapy does for the brain and body. How would you explain it clearly, without jargon?" Ask clients to paraphrase what they have learned so far.

3.3 Domain Two: Metabolism

Every thought, movement, and neurological process depends on energy. Despite comprising roughly 2% of body mass, the brain consumes more than 20% of the body's energy output. After ABI this system is thrown into crisis: neurons are fuel-starved, mitochondrial efficiency drops, inflammation escalates, and oxidative stress compromises structural integrity. In such a state even sophisticated rehabilitation may fall short, like running demanding software on a compromised operating system. If the brain lacks metabolic capacity to sustain therapy, progress stalls before it starts.

Neurometabolic restoration is therefore foundational rather than adjunctive, and it rests on three components.

Mitochondrial health. Mitochondria produce the ATP required for synaptic activity, cognitive processing, and plasticity. After ABI, oxidative stress damages mitochondrial DNA and chronic neuroinflammation depletes mitochondrial resilience, contributing to mental fatigue, poor concentration, and delayed recovery. Cofactors such as CoQ10, NAD+ precursors, alpha-lipoic acid, and PQQ are used clinically to support ATP production, alongside non-pharmacological approaches including photobiomodulation, structured breathwork, and HBOT. *(Evidence label: mitochondrial dysfunction after TBI is well documented (Hiebert et al., 2015). The specific supplement protocols above rest largely on mechanistic rationale rather than ABI outcome trials. HBOT specifically is investigational for chronic mild TBI, with controlled studies not demonstrating benefit beyond sham; see Chapter 3's fuller treatment in the neuroinflammation material.)*

Ketogenic and metabolic strategies. When the injured brain struggles to extract energy from glucose, cognitive symptoms often follow. Ketones provide an alternative fuel that can bypass impaired glucose pathways. Ketogenic diets, exogenous ketones, and strategies such as time-restricted eating are proposed to reduce neuroinflammation and support synaptic repair, with modified low-glycemic protocols or MCT supplementation as gentler options for patients who cannot sustain strict regimens. *(Evidence label: cerebral ketone metabolism after TBI has a genuine mechanistic literature (Prins & Matsumoto, 2014), but human ABI clinical-outcome evidence for ketogenic intervention is limited. Present as reasonable and physiologically grounded, not proven. The originally cited Poff et al. source is unverifiable and has been removed as a citation; the claim is retained as hypothesis-level.)*

Neuroimmune regulation. ABI triggers an inflammatory cascade that, unresolved, becomes a barrier to healing. Overactivated microglia release pro-inflammatory cytokines that disrupt plasticity and cognition, sometimes persisting for months or years. Omega-3 fatty acids, curcumin, and polyphenols such as resveratrol are used to modulate microglial activity, while vagal support, HRV training, and breathwork shift the autonomic system out of chronic sympathetic dominance. When inflammation is better regulated, the brain is more receptive to plastic change. *(Evidence label: microglial biology after TBI is complex rather than uniformly harmful (Loane & Kumar, 2016). HRV biofeedback has reasonable support (Lu et al., 2023); the anti-inflammatory nutraceuticals have general support with limited ABI-specific outcome data, and curcumin's bioavailability constraints apply.)*

3.4 Domain Three: Cognition

Neuroplasticity must be deliberately engaged through structured, targeted input. After ABI, rehabilitation must go beyond rote exercises. The brain adapts to what it repeatedly experiences, so recovery depends on the quality, complexity, and relevance of the stimuli it receives. Repeating movements or drills in isolation is not enough; meaningful outcomes require immersive, multimodal work that mirrors real-world complexity.

Motor learning and dual-task training. In daily life we rarely move in isolation; walking involves processing visual input, making decisions, and managing distraction. Dual-task training challenges the brain to coordinate motor activity with simultaneous cognitive processing, strengthening integration and executive function. Applications include walking while reciting sequences, balancing while problem-solving, or coordinating limb movement while recalling verbal cues. Constraint-induced movement therapy adds plastic demand by encouraging use of the affected limb. *(Evidence label: dual-task and task-specific training have real rehabilitation support, including in stroke populations (Zhang et al., 2022, labeled adjacent-not-ABI); CIMT is well established in stroke with more limited ABI-specific data.)*

Guided visualization and mental rehearsal. Visualizing a task engages pathways overlapping with performing it, which underpins mental rehearsal in stroke, TBI, and ABI recovery. A patient recovering upper-limb function may mentally rehearse grasping a cup, attending to shape, weight, and trajectory. Mirror therapy uses visual feedback from the unaffected limb to engage motor areas associated with the impaired side, and combining these with neuromodulation may enhance motor planning and adaptation. Mental rehearsal also supports memory, planning, and self-efficacy. *(Evidence label: motor imagery and action-observation therapy have a genuine and reasonably developed evidence base (Jackson et al., 2001; Buccino, 2014; Franceschini et al., 2010; Garrison et al., 2010; Hsieh et al., 2020; Rizzolatti & Craighero, 2004), strongest in stroke populations. Hsieh et al. was* *a pilot study in subacute stroke with mixed results across outcome measures; it provides adjacent evidence for the intervention, not direct evidence of effectiveness across ABI populations.)*

Sensory enrichment and multimodal stimulation. The brain learns best when multiple senses are engaged, and multisensory integration reinforces synaptic activity and memory formation. After ABI many patients experience sensory processing difficulty or disconnection from their environment. Rhythmic auditory stimulation and music-based therapy support timing, coordination, and emotional regulation through auditory-motor networks. Tactile interventions support proprioception and body awareness. Olfactory input engages limbic circuitry associated with emotional processing and autobiographical memory. Sensory-enriched environments, designed to engage without overstimulating, can improve attention and learning capacity. *(Evidence label: rhythmic auditory stimulation has reasonable support in gait rehabilitation; broader "sensory enrichment" claims rest largely on animal-model enrichment literature and general principles. Neural Resonance Theory, a recent framework for music-based healing, is a theoretical proposal rather than established clinical evidence.)*

Neuromodulation paired with active therapy. Neurofeedback, entrainment, tDCS, PEMF, and newer protocols such as theta-burst stimulation are most useful when paired with active task-specific movement or cognitive training rather than delivered passively. The pairing is the point: neuromodulation may prime the system, but learning still requires the work.

> **Mind-Body Reflection.** During integrative sessions, subtle shifts occur. Encourage clients to pause afterward and ask: "What felt different today, in my mind, body, or mood?" Reflective awareness supports lasting change.

3.5 Domain Four: Relationship

Relationship-centered care goes beyond compassion; it has measurable physiological effects. When patients feel emotionally safe, heard, and empowered, autonomic regulation shifts in a direction that favors healing. Trust, empathy, and shared decision-making support executive engagement and reduce threat-driven reactivity, creating better conditions for recovery. Trauma-informed communication, simplified educational tools, and consistent emotional support are therapeutic modalities in their own right, not add-ons to therapy.

The clinical substance of this domain, health literacy, teach-back, empathic listening, emotional intelligence, therapeutic presence, is developed fully in Chapter 1 (§1.5) and extended in Chapter 6 and Appendix B. Its place here is to name it as a **target of care**, not merely a manner of delivering care. When a clinician plans an intervention, "which domain am I working in?" should be answerable with Relationship as legitimately as with Metabolism.

Core relational concepts.

- **Relationship-centered care.** The therapeutic bond as an agent of change: empathy, active listening, mutual respect, collaboration. The clinician is a responsive partner, not only a guide.
- **Health literacy and communication.** Translating clinical language into accessible, compassionate terms. Not simplifying content, but connecting through language that meets the patient where they are.
- **Emotional intelligence.** Recognizing and responding to emotional undercurrents, the clinician's own included, which reduces reactivity and increases attunement.
- **Empathic listening and therapeutic presence.** Full presence, with open attention, nonverbal warmth, and curiosity, can support regulation faster than any technique.

Action Step: Relational practice.

- Use everyday language when teaching clinical concepts, inviting questions and pausing to confirm understanding.
- Practice empathic listening: paraphrase concerns, affirm emotional experience, use reflective responses.
- Use teach-back regularly, especially when introducing new tools or home practices, inviting the patient to re-explain in their own words rather than testing recall.
- Attend to nonverbal connection: eye contact, calm vocal tone, open posture, gentle pacing.
- Engage in emotional-intelligence and mindfulness practice as clinician self-care. Regulated practitioners model regulation.

Intervention or practice	Application and frequency	Notes
Empathic listening	Every patient interaction; use reflective responses	Sincerity matters; performed empathy erodes trust
Teach-back method	Each educational session; verify comprehension	Adjust explanations based on what the patient returns

Intervention or practice	Application and frequency	Notes
Emotional intelligence training	Clinician workshops quarterly (2 to 4 hours)	Ongoing practice recommended
Mindful therapeutic presence	Daily clinician practice (10 to 15 minutes)	Integrate into patient sessions, not only personal practice
Patient-friendly communication tools	Visual aids, simplified terminology, continuous use	Customize to the patient's cognitive profile

3.6 Domain Five: Environment

The fifth domain addresses the conditions surrounding the patient: sensory environment, home and clinic design, social support, circadian and light exposure, and the reduction of environmental load that competes with recovery. A nervous system that is chronically overstimulated by noise, lighting, or unpredictable demands has fewer resources available for the work of rehabilitation.

In the original manuscript, the substantive healing-environment content lived primarily in Chapter 6 (Implementation Strategies) and in the environmental-accommodation material now consolidated in Chapter 7 and Appendix C. Rather than duplicate it here, this domain names Environment as a formal target of care and points to its full clinical treatment: **healing environments and sensory accommodation in Chapter 6 and Chapter 7, circadian and light-exposure strategies in Chapter 1 (§1.4, Elimination) and Chapter 5**, and **environmental accessibility guidance in Appendix C**. The domain exists so that environment is planned deliberately rather than left as background.

3.7 Translating the Model into Clinical Practice

The Five Core Domains function as a planning tool. For a given patient, the clinician asks which domains are most disrupted, which are most accessible to intervention right now, and which are being neglected. A patient plateauing in cognitive therapy may need Metabolism addressed before more Cognition work will hold. A patient who cannot tolerate any active intervention may need Relationship and Environment stabilized first. A patient doing well physically but describing loss of self is asking for work that lives in the higher Realms of Chapter 1 and the identity material of Chapter 10.

The Domains answer where. Chapter 9's Three-Phase Model answers when: Priming establishes readiness, Intensive Neural Activation does the demanding work, and Reinforcement consolidates it. Used together, they let a clinician build a plan that is both comprehensive across systems and coherent over time. Neither framework alone is sufficient; a plan that addresses every domain in the wrong order will fail as surely as a well-sequenced plan that ignores metabolic capacity.

CASE EXAMPLE

Priya: Neuroinflammatory and Other Physiologic Contributors

The following is a fictional educational composite based on a commonly encountered clinical pattern, not a specific patient.

Priya was four months out from a concussion when she came in, still living with brain fog and fatigue that hadn't followed the recovery timeline anyone had promised her. Her earlier providers had a ready explanation: depression, or just the frustrating grind of ordinary recovery. Neither one quite fit. The fog had a particular character, worse at certain times of day, more like physical heaviness than low mood, and while her sadness was real, it didn't explain everything she was describing.

Rather than order a broad panel and hope something turned up, the assessment started with what her history actually pointed toward: sleep quality, nutritional adequacy, medication effects, mood, infection history. Any further testing followed from what those areas suggested, not from a hope of finding a hidden answer. What emerged wasn't a single cause. Medical and inflammatory factors were considered where the history suggested they mattered, never assumed present by default, and her emotional distress was treated as neither the whole story nor beside the point.

Care moved on two tracks at once: continued attention to nutrition and sleep, alongside ongoing support for her emotional wellbeing, with neither one taking priority over the other. Over the following weeks, Priya's mental clarity gradually improved and her mood grew somewhat steadier, though she still had days that were noticeably harder than others. It's not possible to say how much of that improvement traced to the physiologic support, the emotional care, the sleep changes, or simply time.

What this composite illustrates is how quickly a premature psychological explanation can obscure a more layered picture, without that meaning the psychological piece was ever unreal. What it cannot establish is a single cause for Priya's symptoms, and it shouldn't be read as evidence that any one factor explains post-concussive brain fog in general.

Chapter 3 Quick-Reference Guide and Summary

Core concepts.

- **Three operating principles:** relationship-centered care, consciousness-based healing, and integrative neuroscience govern how the model is applied.
- **Five Core Domains (where care is directed):** Energy, Metabolism, Cognition, Relationship, Environment.
- **Energy:** neuroelectric stimulation, brainwave optimization, PEMF and photobiomodulation, biofield-based approaches, each at its own evidence level.
- **Metabolism:** mitochondrial health, ketogenic and metabolic strategies, neuroimmune regulation. Foundational, not adjunctive.
- **Cognition:** dual-task training, mental rehearsal and mirror therapy, sensory enrichment, neuromodulation paired with active therapy.
- **Relationship:** a target of care, not only a manner of care.
- **Environment:** named formally here; clinical content in Chapters 6 and 7 and Appendix C.
- **Two frameworks, two questions:** Domains for where, Three-Phase Model (Chapter 9) for when. Neither replaces the other.

Chapter 4: Clinical Protocols for ABI Rehabilitation

Rehabilitation of acquired brain injury is not a one-size-fits-all process. Each patient brings a distinct constellation of symptoms, from cognitive and emotional disruption to metabolic, autonomic, and sensory imbalance. Clinical protocols must be flexible, responsive, and personalized to be effective. This chapter outlines a stepwise approach integrating neuroscience, neuroplasticity-based intervention, frequency-based therapies, and metabolic regulation, with the aim of restoring function while supporting the brain's capacity for repair.

4.1 Stepwise Clinical Assessment

Conventional ABI assessment often falls short. It focuses on structural damage, gross motor impairment, and overt speech deficits, all essential but far from the whole picture. Many survivors experience persistent difficulty that standard tools do not detect: executive dysfunction, brain fog, emotional volatility, autonomic instability, and fatigue can linger for months or years without clear explanation. These often arise from overlooked domains, including cognitive-linguistic processing, autonomic dysregulation, metabolic imbalance, and neuroimmune dysfunction. Without assessing these areas, treatment plans risk addressing surface symptoms while missing what maintains them.

A caution belongs here before the framework itself. The point of a broader assessment is **better-directed** assessment, not more testing by default. Persistent symptoms with unremarkable results in one area do not mean the answer waits in a more specialized test; they may mean a different area is more relevant, or that the symptom is already being managed appropriately without a test result driving that management. Each tier below should be entered because the clinical picture points there, not because it exists.

The Four-Tier ABI Assessment Model

Tier one: cognitive-linguistic and executive function. These skills often go untested in basic neurological exams, yet they shape everyday communication, decision-making, and problem-solving. Standardized instruments assess attention, processing speed, and mental flexibility (for example Trail Making and Stroop), verbal and visual memory and organization (for example the Hopkins Verbal Learning Test, Rey-Osterrieth Complex Figure, and TOMAL-2 for a broader memory profile including delayed recall, working memory, and retention), and language and word-finding (for example Boston Naming Test or CLQT). Metacognitive self-report tools add insight into a patient's awareness of their own difficulties, which strongly affects engagement and goal-setting. Administration and interpretation belong with appropriately qualified clinicians.

Tier two: autonomic function. Dysautonomia after ABI is common, presenting as fatigue, dizziness, poor stress tolerance, and altered heart-rate variability. These symptoms are frequently misattributed to psychological causes when they are rooted in autonomic dysregulation (Mercier et al., 2022). Orthostatic vitals are the practical first step; HRV offers a window into autonomic balance; and formal autonomic testing, including tilt-table testing where indicated, assesses postural stability and responsiveness. Identifying these patterns helps explain the energy crashes and physiological reactivity many patients describe.

Tier three: metabolic and neuroimmune health. Chronic brain fog, low energy, and emotional instability may be driven by inflammation, oxidative stress, or mitochondrial dysfunction. Inflammatory markers such as CRP and IL-6, and measures of redox status, can indicate a chronic inflammatory picture; organic-acid or lactate/pyruvate testing is sometimes used to explore mitochondrial function. Gut-brain evaluation (permeability markers, microbiome composition) may be considered **when the history specifically points there**, not as a default panel. *(Evidence label: these markers describe population-level patterns and general physiology. No single inflammatory or permeability marker diagnoses the cause of an individual patient's persistent post-ABI symptoms, and results should inform rather than dictate care. Several functional-medicine panels in wide clinical use have limited validation for this specific application; Appendix D gives brand-neutral criteria for evaluating any test before ordering it.)*

Tier four: neurophysiological assessment. Quantitative EEG may identify patterns of interest such as excess theta, reduced beta, or disrupted alpha coherence. Two constraints carry through the whole book: qEEG findings are **not specific to TBI** and are influenced by alertness, sleep, medication, psychiatric conditions, and analytic method; and qEEG should **not** independently establish a brain-injury diagnosis, determine severity, or prescribe a neurofeedback protocol. Routine EEG remains clinically established for suspected seizure or episodic altered awareness rather than as a general test for persistent post-concussive symptoms. Neurotransmitter panels are sometimes used to explore dopamine, serotonin, acetylcholine, and GABA status; urinary neurotransmitter testing in particular has significant validity limitations and should not be treated as a direct readout of central nervous system neurotransmitter activity.

Taken together, the four tiers turn assessment from a checklist into a map. Cognitive-linguistic evaluation clarifies how deficits affect independence and quality of life; autonomic testing uncovers hidden contributors to fatigue and stress sensitivity; metabolic and neuroimmune findings identify potential biochemical obstacles; and neurophysiological data describe function over time. Used judiciously, they let clinicians build individualized plans rather than generic ones.

CASE EXAMPLE

Marcus: Autonomic Pattern Recognition

The following is a fictional educational composite, built from patterns commonly seen in clinical practice, not a specific patient.

Two providers had already told Marcus his symptoms were anxiety. He wasn't convinced. Eight months out from a moderate traumatic brain injury in a car accident, he was dealing with dizziness on standing, fatigue that came and went without warning, and a racing heart he couldn't tie to any obvious trigger. He'd been offered anti-anxiety medication and declined it, unsure it actually matched what he was living with.

He wasn't wrong to be uncertain. The dizziness had a clear postural signature, worse standing, easing when he sat, that didn't map neatly onto anxiety alone, even though anxiety was genuinely part of the picture too. Orthostatic vital signs went into his workup as the primary tool for assessing this, with heart rate variability monitoring added later as something he could track himself, not as a stand-in for the formal assessment. His emotional state stayed part of the conversation the whole time; it didn't get set aside the moment a physiological pattern showed up.

The postural pattern in his vitals fit autonomic involvement, a recognized feature after brain injury, though how often it actually occurs varies across the research and shouldn't be assumed for any one patient. None of this ruled out anxiety. The two plausibly feed each other: an unpredictable body is itself anxiety-provoking, and heightened arousal can worsen autonomic symptoms in turn. So the plan addressed both together rather than picking a single explanation.

Treatment started with what was accessible and easy to monitor: breath practice, hydration, electrolyte attention, adjusted for his blood pressure, kidney function, and medications rather than applied as one fixed amount for everyone. Body scanning helped him build interoceptive awareness, though it doesn't work for everyone the same way, and some people find it intensifies distress instead of easing it. HRV biofeedback came later, once there was a clear question it was meant to answer and a way to track whether it was actually helping.

Over several months, Marcus's dizziness episodes became more predictable to him. He learned to catch early signals and use a regulation tool before things escalated, and his anxiety about his body's unpredictability eased, though it never disappeared entirely. He still had symptomatic days, especially after poor sleep or overexertion, and he hadn't returned to his pre-injury activity baseline.

This composite illustrates a common pattern: dysautonomia and anxiety coexisting and reinforcing each other after brain injury, where treating the physiological pattern doesn't mean dismissing the emotional one. It doesn't demonstrate that HRV biofeedback or any specific tool caused Marcus's improvement, and his experience doesn't predict another patient's outcome.

4.2 Neuroplasticity-Driven Rehabilitation Protocols

Neuroplasticity is the mechanism through which functional improvement occurs, but it does not happen automatically. It requires the right environment, the right stimulation, and the right timing. The QIM model applies a three-phase approach to activating and sustaining it. This is the same **Three-Phase Model** developed in Chapter 9; introduced here in its clinical-protocol form, it is presented as the author's original translational synthesis for sequencing ABI care, with individual components carrying their own evidence labels.

Phase one: priming the brain for plasticity. If neurotransmitter systems are dysregulated or the brain is inflamed or metabolically depleted, capacity for plastic change is limited. Priming aims to establish readiness. Aerobic exercise is included in guideline recommendations for persistent post-concussion symptoms, although the recommendations are weak and based on low to very low certainty evidence (Rytter et al., 2021). GABAergic and inhibitory balance may be supported through magnesium-based strategies, mindfulness practice, and entrainment tools (Slutsky et al., 2010; Tang et al., 2007, both non-ABI populations). Cerebral oxygenation approaches include breathwork and photobiomodulation, with HBOT investigational rather than established for chronic mild TBI.

> **Important evidence correction.** The original chapter recommended citicoline and L-tyrosine as priming agents for dopaminergic and cholinergic support. **Citicoline was tested directly in TBI in the COBRIT trial** (Zafonte et al., 2012, n=1213), the largest and most rigorous trial to date, and **did not show benefit**. That negative finding is retained and stated plainly here rather than omitted. L-tyrosine and related catecholaminergic strategies remain a plausible hypothesis based on general neuropharmacology, without dedicated ABI trial support, and are labeled as hypothesis rather than recommendation. The original bundled citation (Foster et al.; McMorris et al.) did not support the ABI-specific claim as written and has been unbundled accordingly.

Phase two: intensive neural activation. This stage delivers targeted, repetitive, multisensory input to drive functional change. Action-observation and mirror-based approaches have patients observe and imitate goal-directed behavior, engaging circuits involved in action understanding and motor planning; these have a reasonably developed evidence base, strongest in stroke populations (Buccino, 2014; Franceschini et al., 2010; Garrison et al., 2010; Hsieh et al., 2020; Rizzolatti & Craighero, 2004). Hsieh et al. was a pilot study in subacute stroke with mixed results across outcome measures, offering adjacent evidence rather than direct evidence of effectiveness across ABI populations. Dual-task training integrates cognitive and motor demand, reflecting real-world function; supporting evidence includes stroke-population work labeled adjacent-not-ABI (Zhang et al., 2022). Guided visualization and mental rehearsal engage overlapping pathways to physical execution, useful when overt performance is limited (Jackson et al., 2001, correctly dated; the original manuscript's 2003 date was an error).

Phase three: reinforcement and neuromodulation. The goal here is to stabilize and integrate gains. Neurofeedback and entrainment are used to support sustained regulation of arousal, focus, and emotional state (Gruzelier, 2014; see also Cicerone et al., 2019 for evidence-based cognitive rehabilitation more broadly). This phase emphasizes **generalization**: skills learned in clinic must transfer to daily life through real-world task integration such as cooking, navigating public spaces, or managing routines, consistent with motor-learning principles of relevance, variability, and context (Kleim & Jones, 2008). Metacognitive strategy training supports self-monitoring and sustained engagement (Kennedy et al., 2008), helping patients participate actively rather than receive care passively.

> **Clinician Tip: Introducing PEMF.** Start at the lowest intensity and increase gradually. Many ABI patients are sensitive to frequency-based tools, so pacing matters. Monitor for overstimulation or rebound fatigue.

4.3 Frequency Therapies: PEMF, Light, and Vagus Nerve

ABI disrupts the structural and chemical integrity of the brain, and its rhythmic signaling as well. When coherence is lost, brain fog, emotional dysregulation, fatigue, and autonomic instability often follow. Frequency-based tools aim to stabilize the nervous system and create conditions more receptive to plastic change. They are not replacements for cognitive or physical rehabilitation; they are groundwork that can make those therapies more effective.

Vagus nerve support targets the primary parasympathetic pathway to support regulation and homeostasis. ABI often suppresses vagal tone, favoring sympathetic dominance that impedes recovery. Accessible interventions include slow diaphragmatic breathing, humming, cold exposure, and, where available and appropriate, transcutaneous vagus nerve stimulation. Combined with HRV biofeedback, these can support stress tolerance and emotional regulation (Lu et al., 2023, HRV biofeedback; Breit et al., 2018, vagal modulation of brain-body signaling). For patients with dysautonomia, sleep disruption, or persistent post-injury anxiety, these are among the most practical tools available. *(Evidence label: implanted VNS is an established therapy for specific epilepsy and depression indications and should not be conflated with non-invasive tVNS or breath-based vagal support, which have far more limited evidence.)*

PEMF therapy delivers low-frequency electromagnetic pulses studied for effects on mitochondrial activity, inflammatory signaling, and autonomic measures including HRV. It is used clinically for cognitive fatigue and autonomic dysregulation. *(Evidence label: emerging. Supporting literature is substantially mechanistic, preclinical, or from adjacent populations; ABI-specific controlled human evidence remains limited. The original chapter specified "10 Hz, 20 to 30 minutes, 3 to 5 times weekly" as a validated protocol. That specificity is not supported by the current evidence base and has been reframed: parameters vary widely across devices and studies, should start conservatively, and must be individualized with attention to sensitivity and rebound fatigue.)*

Photobiomodulation uses red and near-infrared light to target mitochondrial cytochrome c oxidase, supporting ATP synthesis and oxygen utilization while reducing oxidative stress. Applications include transcranial delivery for cognition, mood, and sleep. *(Evidence label: promising, with the most developed mechanistic rationale in this group, but resting largely on small studies, including a frequently cited pair of chronic-TBI case reports (Naeser et al., 2011). Not an established standard.)*

> **Teach-Back Tool.** "If a friend asked what PEMF or neurofeedback is, how would you explain it simply?"

4.4 Gut-Brain and Immune Restoration Protocols

The gut and brain communicate bidirectionally, influencing cognition, inflammation, and emotional regulation. After ABI this communication is often disrupted, contributing to persistent neuroinflammation, fatigue, brain fog, and mood instability. Gut health is rarely the focus of conventional neurorehabilitation, yet it participates in immune regulation and neurotransmitter balance.

ABI is associated with dysbiosis, which can weaken intestinal barrier integrity and allow inflammatory compounds such as lipopolysaccharide into circulation, potentially contributing to neuroinflammation that interferes with repair. Addressing this cycle is a reasonable component of care.

Polyphenols including curcumin, resveratrol, and EGCG are used to modulate inflammatory signaling in both gut and brain. Curcumin's poor natural bioavailability is clinically decisive: piperine-enhanced, phytosome, or nanoparticle formulations are needed to reach meaningful levels, which changes whether a recommendation works at all.

Barrier support may include L-glutamine, zinc carnosine, colostrum, and polyphenol-rich foods, alongside microbiome support with targeted probiotics and prebiotic fiber. *(The original chapter specified "10 to 50 billion CFU/day." Probiotic effects are strain-specific rather than dose-generic, so CFU counts alone are a poor guide; strain selection, indication, and tolerance matter more, and introduction should be gradual given GI sensitivity in this population.)*

Essential fatty acids, particularly EPA and DHA, support membrane integrity and inflammation resolution, and attention to the omega-3 to omega-6 ratio through diet or supplementation is a reasonable foundational step.

> **Evidence label for this section.** The gut-brain axis is well established as biology (Carabotti et al., 2015; Cryan et al., 2019, both general reviews). Evidence that microbiome-directed treatment improves **ABI recovery specifically** is limited (Pathare et al., 2020, with its own human-study limitations). "Leaky gut" and LPS-mediated neuroinflammation are mechanistically plausible and actively researched rather than clinically confirmed pathways in ABI. Present gut-supportive care as reasonable, low-risk, and foundational, not as proven ABI treatment.
>
> **Teach-Back Tool.** "Can you explain how gut health affects the brain, and share one food or habit that supports both?"

4.5 A Guiding Framework for Clinical Integration

What follows is a flexible framework rather than a fixed protocol. It invites clinicians to explore integrative strategies supporting neurological, metabolic, emotional, and regulatory recovery, adapted to each client's presentation, readiness, and pace. Use it as a map, not a mandate.

Comprehensive assessment

- **Clinical interview and history.** Explore injury history, symptom onset, and the client's own understanding of their difficulties. Include structured tools for cognitive-emotional status and screening for co-occurring trauma or stress-related patterns.

- **Neurometabolic evaluation.** Targeted functional testing may assess inflammation, nutrient status, and mitochondrial or oxidative markers, ordered from the history rather than as a broad default screen.
- **Neurological and regulatory assessment.** qEEG may offer insight into cortical dysregulation within the constraints named in §4.1. HRV provides a dynamic snapshot of autonomic balance and is among the most practical repeatable measures available.
- **Functional and cognitive-linguistic profiling.** Assess communication, memory, attention, executive function, and motor integration with standardized, observation-based tools. This forms the foundation for goal-oriented, personalized rehabilitation.

Core domains of intervention

These map directly onto the Five Core Domains of Chapter 3.

- **Neurometabolic optimization (Metabolism).** Support metabolic function through food-based approaches (anti-inflammatory, lower-glycemic) and mitochondrial cofactors. The intent is not to "fix" with supplements but to build the metabolic resilience that lets plasticity occur.
- **Bioelectromagnetic regulation (Energy).** Where clinicians have appropriate training and equipment, PEMF or neurofeedback may be introduced to support autonomic tone and coherence. Parameters must always be adjusted to the patient's response.
- **Neuroplasticity activation (Cognition).** Dual-task training, mental imagery, and movement-based integration help engage disrupted pathways. Sessions should be engaging, safe, and progressively layered. Mental rehearsal is especially useful for those with fatigue or mobility limitations.
- **Gut-brain axis support (Metabolism/Form).** Phased interventions to support gut resilience, introduced mindfully to avoid overstimulation.
- **Consciousness-based and emotional healing (Relationship/Awareness).** Mindfulness, guided visualization, and breathwork support regulation and self-awareness. Some clients benefit from formal therapeutic support to process trauma and rebuild narrative identity after injury.

Monitoring and adaptive planning

- **Ongoing reassessment.** Periodic check-ins and re-testing help track progress and adjust plans. Domains worth revisiting include cognition, sleep quality, emotional regulation, GI status, and overall energy.
- **Biofeedback and nervous-system data.** Review of HRV trends, neurofeedback data, and patient-submitted metrics can guide pacing and therapeutic load.
- **Patient reflection and journaling.** Symptom logs and reflective entries build insight, inform progression, and strengthen the therapeutic alliance. Tools for this are provided in Appendix A.

> **Teach-Back Tool.** Provide a one-page tracker titled "What I Notice," with simple daily check-ins for sleep, mood, memory, energy, and digestion, plus a notes area. Encourage clients to bring it to each session.

Integrative tools in practice

Rather than prescriptive formulas, the QIM approach encourages clinicians to understand the reasoning behind each modality so they can think critically and adapt. The tools below are possibilities to explore with discernment.

Neurofeedback supports regulation of brainwave activity, with applications for emotional regulation, cognitive performance, and sleep stability. It is particularly relevant for clients struggling with anxiety, impulsivity, or poor focus. Formal practice requires equipment and certification; clinicians can begin by understanding brainwave dynamics and client readiness. **Board certification through BCIA (Biofeedback Certification International Alliance)** is the recognized credentialing pathway for biofeedback and neurofeedback, and **EEGInfo** provides clinical training and protocol education. **NeurOptimal** is one widely used dynamical neurofeedback system suited to clinic or supervised home use. These are named as examples of the training and equipment landscape rather than as endorsements; pursue board-recognized certification rather than device-specific vendor training alone, since a credential tied to one manufacturer does not transfer.

Nutritional support. Targeted nutrients such as mitochondrial cofactors, magnesium, and omega-3s are commonly depleted after brain injury or chronic stress. Supplementation should be based on the individual's presentation, available labs, and clinical observation rather than protocol defaults. Appendix D provides brand-neutral quality standards for evaluating any supplement: third-party testing, verified potency, absence of undisclosed ingredients, and transparent sourcing.

Gut-brain support. May include probiotics, prebiotics, digestive enzymes, L-glutamine, or anti-inflammatory nutrition, aiming to support barrier integrity and vagal signaling.

Mindfulness and somatic awareness. Restoring present-moment awareness through breath, movement, or quiet reflection supports self-regulation and vagal tone. Mindfulness need not mean sitting still; it may look like painting, walking barefoot, or holding a warm cup of tea with intention.

Healing unfolds at the speed of safety, and the clinician's presence is part of what makes it possible.

Chapter 4 Quick-Reference Guide and Summary

Core concepts.

- **Four-Tier Assessment Model:** cognitive-linguistic and executive function; autonomic function; metabolic and neuroimmune health; neurophysiological assessment. Enter each tier because the clinical picture points there, not by default.
- **Three-phase neuroplasticity protocol:** priming, intensive neural activation, reinforcement and generalization. Citicoline's negative COBRIT result is stated plainly; L-tyrosine is labeled hypothesis.
- **Frequency therapies:** vagal support and HRV work (most practical), PEMF (emerging), photobiomodulation (promising, small studies). Implanted VNS is not equivalent to non-invasive vagal support.
- **Gut-brain and immune restoration:** reasonable, low-risk, foundational care rather than proven ABI treatment. Curcumin bioavailability and probiotic strain-specificity are the clinically decisive details.
- **Integration framework:** assessment, five-domain intervention, and adaptive monitoring, mapped to Chapter 3's Domains and Chapter 9's Phases.

Practical clinical actions.

- Assess across all four tiers as the presentation warrants, and document what each tier is meant to answer before ordering it.
- Introduce frequency-based tools at conservative starting parameters, individualized and monitored, rather than at fixed protocol settings.
- Integrate dual-task cognitive-motor work into routine rehabilitation, matching challenge to current capacity.
- Apply gut-supportive strategies gradually, watching GI tolerance, with strain-appropriate rather than dose-generic probiotic selection.
- Build mindfulness and emotional processing into care routinely, tailoring technique and duration to cognitive capacity.

Intervention	Common use patterns	Considerations
PEMF therapy	Often integrated into sessions multiple times per week	Begin gently; observe for sensory sensitivity and rebound fatigue; parameters individualized, not fixed
Neurofeedback	Implemented as part of a structured neurotraining plan	Requires training and certification; regular monitoring and calibration essential; qEEG alone does not prescribe protocol
Nutritional support	May include mitochondrial or cognition-targeted nutrients	Consider baseline labs; track change over time; brand-neutral quality criteria in Appendix D
Gut-brain optimization	Dietary strategies and microbiome support	Introduce gradually; watch GI tolerance; strain-specific selection
Mindfulness practice	Daily or routine practice	Tailor technique and length to cognitive capacity
Dual-task training	Movement combined with cognitive demand	Match challenge to ability; increase complexity gradually

Chapter 5: Case-Based Applications

5.1 Reframing Recovery: The Power of Personalized Protocols

Acquired brain injury is never a linear condition, and neither is its recovery. Each person's healing is shaped by a distinct mix of neurological deficits, systemic imbalances, personal history, and environment. Conventional rehabilitation often emphasizes functional restoration through standardized protocols; recovery tends to happen when treatment is personalized, adaptive, and integrative.

This chapter shows how QIM principles are applied across a whole recovery arc, using extended case material to make abstract frameworks concrete. Individual episodes from these cases appear alongside the clinical chapters they illustrate (Chapters 3, 4, 5, 6, 7, 9, and 10); this chapter gathers the reasoning that connects them.

5.2 How to Read the Composite Cases

Every case in this book is a fictional educational composite based on commonly encountered clinical patterns. No composite is a real patient or a real treatment record. Each is written to illustrate a pattern of clinical reasoning, and each states its own limits: what the pattern illustrates, and what it cannot establish.

This matters for how you use them. A composite can show you how a clinician thinks through a confusing presentation, how sequencing decisions get made, or how a premature explanation can obscure a fuller picture. A composite cannot serve as evidence that an intervention works, cannot establish causation, and cannot tell you what proportion of patients respond. Where this book makes claims about effectiveness, those claims rest on the cited literature and its evidence labels, never on the cases.

The three recurring composites are:

- **Marcus**, whose arc runs from autonomic pattern recognition (Chapter 4), through gastrointestinal symptoms considered within a broader recovery picture (Chapter 6), to sequencing and integration across his whole course of care (Chapter 9).
- **Priya**, whose arc runs from neuroinflammatory and other physiologic contributors (Chapter 3) to a closer look at hormonal and metabolic function (Chapter 5).
- **Theo**, whose arc runs from trauma-informed engagement (Chapter 7) to identity integration over the long arc of recovery (Chapter 10).

Following one person across several chapters is deliberate. It shows what a fragmented, episode-by-episode view cannot: that the same patient is simultaneously a metabolic story, an autonomic story, a relational story, and an identity story, and that which one you are looking at depends on which question you are asking.

CASE EXAMPLE

Priya, Continued: A Closer Look at Hormonal and Metabolic Function

Priya's composite story continues, the same fictional educational composite, not a real patient.

A few months later, Priya's brain fog had eased, but her fatigue hadn't, and now there was irregular sleep and a menstrual cycle that had changed since her injury. Her earlier bloodwork, a basic metabolic panel and thyroid screen, had come back within normal range, and that had been treated as closing the question. But normal by what measure? The panel had never been positioned to catch what might actually be happening, and the persistence of her symptoms despite "normal" results was itself worth taking seriously.

A more targeted evaluation followed, one that accounted for where she was in her cycle when tested, her medications, and the narrow scope of the original panel. Her cycle changes specifically prompted a referral for medical and gynecologic evaluation rather than a general adjustment to her existing care. Whatever that evaluation found was read alongside her broader symptoms and history, not treated as a diagnosis on its own; nothing here rested on the assumption that menstrual changes alone proved post-injury hormonal dysfunction. A normal initial screen doesn't close a door. It can simply mean more history, more monitoring, or a more specific test is warranted, not that a hidden answer is sitting somewhere waiting to be uncovered.

Care moved forward from there: the gynecologic follow-up, sleep- and cycle-related attention, layered onto the nutritional and emotional-support work already underway from her earlier care. Over the following months, her sleep gradually stabilized and her energy grew somewhat more consistent, though it's not possible to credit any single piece of that to one intervention. Her fatigue never fully resolved, and untangling how much came from the gynecologic follow-up versus everything else already in motion isn't something this case can do.

What this shows is that a normal panel doesn't mean nothing physiologically relevant is happening; timing, scope, and context all shape what a test can actually detect. What it doesn't show is that conventional reference ranges are generally inadequate, and no specific biomarker value here should be read as representative or diagnostic.

5.3 What the Cases Are Meant to Teach

That the presenting explanation is often incomplete without being wrong. Priya's arc begins with providers attributing her persistent fog and fatigue to depression or ordinary recovery. Neither explanation is dismissed as false; her sadness is real. The clinical work is recognizing that a real explanation can still be partial, and that pursuing the fuller picture does not require declaring the first one wrong.

That assessment should follow the history rather than sweep broadly. In Priya's case, evaluation starts from what her history actually points toward, sleep quality, nutritional adequacy, medication effects, mood, infection history, with further testing following from what those areas suggest rather than from hope that something will turn up. This is the Chapter 4 assessment principle in narrative form.

That order matters as much as content. Marcus's arc, read end to end, looks like a deliberate structure rather than a pile of interventions: foundational, low-burden work first, then more active regulation tools, then later additions once he had capacity for them. This is the Three-Phase Model made visible. It is also where the honest limit lives: no single composite can establish how much the sequencing itself contributed versus the individual components or simply time.

That recovery is eventually an identity question. Theo's arc moves from the early work of establishing enough safety to engage at all, to something that no functional scale captures well: who he understands himself to be after injury. Chapter 10 takes this up directly.

5.4 Practitioner FAQs

Clinicians applying this material in practice tend to ask the same practical questions.

"How do I integrate QIM techniques into a conventional rehabilitation program?" Start small and build. Layer one or two integrative interventions onto existing plans rather than restructuring everything. If you already run standard PT/OT sessions, introduce a brief HRV breathing practice at the start, or discuss anti-inflammatory nutrition alongside existing work. Explain to the patient and the team why you are adding it, for instance that breath-based regulation supports readiness so that therapy lands better. Over time, methods that demonstrate value become routine.

"What if a patient is skeptical about energy-based therapy or meditation?" Meet patients where they are, and lead with mechanism and outcomes rather than framing. Neurofeedback is accurately described as brainwave biofeedback training for attention and regulation; mindfulness is accurately described as attention and emotion-regulation training. Neither description requires spiritual or energetic language, and both are more honest about what the evidence supports. Invite a short trial and track results together. Skepticism is also reasonable, and a patient who declines a modality should not be treated as noncompliant.

"How can I measure progress objectively with an integrative approach?" Use standard neuropsychological and functional measures as the backbone, then add repeatable measures from the integrative toolkit: HRV for autonomic trends, symptom and function tracking (Appendix A), sleep and fatigue measures, and where clinically indicated, inflammatory markers. Be honest about what each measure can support: HRV trends describe autonomic state, not recovery globally, and qEEG changes are not by themselves evidence of clinical improvement.

"I have limited time with patients. How do I fit this in?" Be strategic rather than comprehensive. Start with one cornerstone habit likely to produce cascading benefit; sleep and a brief daily regulation practice are usually the highest-yield candidates. Group-based delivery works well for breath and regulation training. Home practice and simple tracking tools extend care beyond the visit without extending your session time.

5.5 Case-Guided Clinical Integration Reference

The table below offers flexible therapeutic domains rather than fixed doses or durations. Adapt based on functional testing, symptom feedback, and therapeutic response. Use it as a compass, not a formula. Domains map to the Five Core Domains of Chapter 3.

Therapeutic domain	Guiding applications	Clinical considerations
Neurometabolic support (Metabolism)	Mitochondrial cofactors and omega-3s may support energy availability	Adjust based on testing and fatigue patterns; foundational rather than curative; evidence largely mechanistic for ABI
Energetic and frequency therapies (Energy)	PEMF and related tools may support regulation and coherence	Apply only with proper training; start conservatively and individualize; emerging evidence base
Neurofeedback and brain training (Energy/Cognition)	Neurofeedback protocols to support emotional regulation and cortical balance	Reassess periodically to stay aligned with the evolving picture; qEEG alone does not prescribe protocol

Therapeutic domain	Guiding applications	Clinical considerations
Gut-brain interventions (Metabolism)	Probiotics, prebiotics, glutamine, anti-inflammatory nutrition	Introduce slowly; monitor for GI discomfort, histamine sensitivity, or cognitive shifts; strain-specific selection
Dual-task neuroplasticity (Cognition)	Movement-cognition integration, for example walking plus recall	Modify complexity based on fatigue, motor ability, and attention
Emotional resilience practices (Relationship/Awareness)	Mindfulness, breathwork, guided imagery, visualization	Tailor frequency and intensity to cognitive tolerance and emotional safety; screen for trauma activation

Caution: Supplement Interactions. Before recommending herbal or adaptogenic supplements, check for drug interactions. Botanicals including Ginkgo, Ashwagandha, and Rhodiola can affect blood pressure, anticoagulation, or neurotransmitter activity. Dose conservatively and coordinate with prescribing clinicians.

Clinician Tip: Translate Lab Data into Food Choices. Do not just explain lab results; personalize them. Link a low omega-3 index to a specific meal, or a B12 concern to specific foods. Food-based examples build understanding and long-term health literacy.

Mind-Body Reflection: Teaching Through the Senses. Are you attuned to how noise, lighting, scent, and pace affect your clients' capacity to learn and engage? What assumptions do you hold about attention, clarity, or memory? How might you adapt your environment or delivery for sensory-sensitive clients?

Chapter 5 Quick-Reference Guide and Summary

Core concepts.

- **Disclosed composites, not case reports.** All case material is fictional educational composite, clearly labeled, carrying no invented statistics and no claim to published-evidence status.
- **Recurring cast across chapters.** Marcus (autonomic, GI, sequencing), Priya (neuroinflammatory, hormonal-metabolic), Theo (trauma-informed engagement, identity).
- **What cases can and cannot do.** They illustrate reasoning; they do not establish efficacy, causation, or response rates.

- **Individualization over protocol.** Assessment follows history; intervention follows assessment; sequencing follows capacity.
- **Practitioner FAQs** address integration into conventional settings, patient skepticism, honest outcome measurement, and time constraints.

Chapter 6: Implementation Strategies for Clinicians

6.1 Introduction: Where to Begin

Integrating Quantum Integrative Medicine into ABI rehabilitation offers opportunity, and yet most clinicians who find the ideas compelling still hesitate at the threshold. The hesitation is not usually about whether the concepts are sound. It is about Monday morning. You have a caseload, documentation requirements, productivity expectations, and a team that did not ask to change how it practices. Where, exactly, does any of this fit?

That question deserves a serious answer rather than encouragement. ABI rehabilitation is already complex and interdisciplinary. Adding frequency-based therapies, metabolic interventions, and consciousness-informed practice on top of an existing workload can feel like being handed a second job. Some clinicians anticipate institutional resistance and are usually right to. Others worry that patients accustomed to conventional rehabilitation will find this strange, and some will. How can any of this be incorporated into insurance-based rehabilitation centers, private practices, or telehealth models without an overhaul nobody has authorized?

The answer running through this chapter is that you do not implement a model. You implement one intervention, with one patient population, and you watch what happens. The clinicians who successfully shift their practice almost never do it by adopting a framework wholesale. They do it by finding that a five-minute breathing practice at the start of a session makes the next forty minutes more productive, and then wondering what else might be true.

This chapter provides the roadmap: how to structure a program, how to match interventions to the phase of recovery a patient is actually in, how to build interdisciplinary collaboration that is real rather than nominal, how to educate patients whose injury has affected the very capacities education depends on, how to design environments that support rather than tax the nervous system, how to use language and coaching as clinical tools, which digital and assistive technologies earn their place, and how to work through the practical barriers of cost, skepticism, and institutional inertia.

A word about how to read the recommendations. Some of what follows has strong evidence, some is reasonable and low-risk, and some is common practice with limited support. The chapter labels these as it goes, because a clinician deciding what to try on Monday needs to know which category a suggestion falls into. Confidence you have not earned is the fastest way to lose a skeptical colleague, and the fastest way to fail a patient who trusted the confidence.

6.2 Building a QIM-Based ABI Rehabilitation Program

Conventional approaches tend to treat symptoms in isolation, dividing care into physical therapy, speech-language therapy, and cognitive rehabilitation. Each of these matters enormously. The problem is not the disciplines; it is that they frequently operate in parallel rather than in concert, so that nobody is asking whether the patient's metabolic state, autonomic regulation, and sleep are undermining everything the disciplines are trying to accomplish.

A QIM-based program is built on four layers. The layering is not decorative. It reflects a clinical judgment about sequence: the lower layers create the physiological conditions that make the upper layers possible, and skipping them is the most common reason good rehabilitation stalls.

Neurometabolic optimization provides the biochemical foundation. ABI disrupts mitochondrial function, destabilizes neuroimmune regulation, and can sustain chronic inflammation for months or years. This layer addresses nutrition, mitochondrial cofactors, anti-inflammatory support, and blood-sugar stability. The reasoning is simple: neuroplastic change is metabolically expensive. A brain that cannot reliably produce ATP cannot do the work of rewiring, no matter how well designed the therapy that asks it to. When a patient plateaus despite excellent therapy, this layer is where I would look first.

Neuroplasticity-driven rehabilitation engages the brain's capacity to reorganize through structured, repetitive, purposeful intervention: action-observation and mirror-based work, dual-task cognitive-motor training, guided visualization, and neurofeedback. What distinguishes this from generic exercise is specificity and relevance. The brain adapts to what it repeatedly does, so the practice must resemble what the patient actually needs to do. Repetition of an abstract task builds skill at that abstract task and often nothing else.

Bioelectromagnetic regulation addresses electrical coherence and autonomic rhythm through PEMF, photobiomodulation, and vagal support, each at the evidence level established in Chapters 2 through 4. This layer is the most variable in its support and should be introduced with the clearest labeling. HRV-based work sits at the strong end; PEMF and photobiomodulation are emerging; the more speculative frequency tools are optional adjuncts rather than program requirements.

Consciousness and relationship-centered healing addresses belief, trauma, meaning, and relational safety. Guided practice, trauma-informed care, language-based reframing, and mental training help patients reconnect with their own resources. This layer is often treated as the soft one, which gets it backwards. A patient who does not feel safe will not engage the demanding work in the layers above, and a clinician who cannot establish that safety will find that their technical excellence does not transfer.

Woven through all four is **patient empowerment**. QIM emphasizes self-directed neuroplasticity, and the practical expression of that is what happens between sessions. An hour of therapy a week is roughly one percent of a patient's waking life. The remaining ninety-nine percent is where recovery is won or lost, which is why home programs, tracking tools, and patient education are not adjuncts to the clinical work. They are most of it.

Why start with the metabolic and regulatory layers. Beginning here is deliberate and worth stating plainly, because it runs against the instinct to lead with the most interesting tool. Foundational supports calm inflammation, support cellular energy, and improve autonomic regulation. They are also inexpensive, low-risk, and unlikely to provoke a turf argument with a skeptical colleague. Sleep, hydration, pacing, light exposure, and breath-based regulation cost nothing and can be started this week. If you implement nothing else from this book, implement those, and you will have captured a substantial portion of the available benefit.

> **Action Step.** Select one primary intervention, nutritional support, a regulation practice, or a neuroplasticity approach, and map a two-week trial plan for a small number of patients. Keep it simple, measurable, and individualized. Track changes in sleep, mood, cognition, and somatic symptoms. Two weeks is long enough to see signal and short enough that abandoning it costs nothing.

6.3 Structuring the Patient Journey

Recovery from ABI is anything but predictable. Some days patients feel progress; other days they are flattened by fatigue, groping for words, unable to hold a thought. This cycle is frustrating and entirely normal, and one of the more useful things a clinician can do is say so out loud, early, before the patient concludes that a bad week means they are going backwards.

Patients often arrive believing recovery should be a straight line, and the belief itself causes harm. Neuroplasticity does not work that way. It moves in waves, through bursts of progress, plateaus, and setbacks that frequently follow periods of gain. The clinical task is not to eliminate this variability but to work with it, matching what we ask of the nervous system to what it can currently deliver.

Phase one: acute recovery (roughly 0 to 3 months)

The first months can feel like being lost in fog. Patients describe relentless fatigue, sensory overload, memory lapses, and emotional swings that arrive without warning. Many describe feeling that the lights are on but the processing is happening somewhere far away.

The instinct in conventional rehabilitation is to begin therapy promptly, and for good reason: early mobilization matters, and in many conditions delay costs function. But in a nervous system that is metabolically depleted and inflammatorily active, pushing cognitive or physical demand too early can backfire in a way that costs weeks. Patients who crash learn that effort produces punishment, and that lesson is difficult to unlearn.

The focus in this phase belongs on stabilization: reducing inflammatory load, supporting energy production, and regulating autonomic function through breathwork, HRV-guided practice, and gentle vagal support. These are not dramatic interventions and they do not look impressive in a note. Without them, patients burn out early and arrive at the phase where meaningful gains are possible with nothing left to spend.

What this looks like practically. Establish a consistent wake time and morning light exposure. Address hydration and electrolytes, which are commonly neglected and easily corrected. Support sleep aggressively, including screening for sleep-disordered breathing, which is common after brain injury and specifically treatable. Introduce brief daily regulation practice, two to five minutes, at a time already anchored in the patient's routine. Educate the family that doing less now is not giving up; it is the thing that makes later work possible. Defer high-demand cognitive and physical rehabilitation until fatigue crashes and autonomic instability begin to settle.

> **Clinician Tip.** Before initiating conventional rehabilitation protocols, ask a question that sounds simple and is not: "Is this brain ready to receive therapy?" Assess whether the patient is experiencing post-exertional crashes or sensory overwhelm, whether signs of dysautonomia are interfering with function, and whether inflammation, sleep, and energy metabolism have been addressed. Use this phase to stabilize before stimulating. Reframing rest as active neuro-support, rather than as absence of treatment, is often the most therapeutic move available early on, and it is one families need help understanding.
>
> **A caution on dosing language.** The original manuscript specified supplement doses for this phase. Those have been reframed as clinician-guided and individualized, because the evidence does not support fixed dosing protocols in this population and because supplement decisions in the acute phase interact with medications, medical status, and clinical instability in ways that make protocol thinking inappropriate. Ranges that are well supported appear in Appendix E with their context.

Phase two: subacute neurorehabilitation (roughly 3 to 12 months)

By around three months the fog often begins to lift. Patients tolerate more stimulation, sustain focus longer, and start to recognize themselves again. This is where the substantive neuroplasticity work belongs, and where the most durable gains are typically made.

Greater responsiveness does not mean stability. Many patients in this phase experience an exhausting alternation of good and bad days that they, and often their families, interpret as random. It is rarely random. It usually tracks cumulative load across the preceding two or three days, which is precisely what makes tracking useful here.

Think of this phase as training rather than healing. The nervous system is relearning how to function, and like any learning process it requires repetition, progressive challenge, and recovery between efforts. The clinical art is calibration: enough demand to drive adaptation, not so much that the patient spends the following two days recovering from the session.

Deepen the neuroplasticity work. Neurofeedback, action-observation and mirror therapy, and progressive cognitive retraining belong here, delivered with enough intensity and specificity to matter. This is also where dual-task work earns its place, because real-world function is almost always dual-task.

Manage energy and sensory load deliberately. Structured pacing with rest taken *before* fatigue rather than after is the single most useful principle in this phase. Patients naturally push until they crash, then rest until they feel able, then push again, which produces the boom-and-bust pattern that stalls recovery. Interrupting that cycle often produces more progress than adding any intervention.

Continue metabolic support as demand increases, since the energetic cost of this phase is higher than the last.

> **Clinician Tip.** Do not confuse functional tolerance with full recovery. Patients often present as sharper in this phase while their reserves remain thin. Ask whether post-exertional worsening is following sessions, whether readiness is actually being measured rather than assumed, and whether intensity matches metabolic and emotional capacity. Encourage a train, recover, reassess rhythm. Treat a bad day as information about load rather than as regression, and say that to the patient explicitly, because they will otherwise read it as failure.

Phase three: long-term recovery and optimization (12 months and beyond)

By the one-year mark many patients have regained a workable version of ordinary life. They are back at work, re-engaged with relationships, functioning. This is not the finish line, and it is also not a guarantee of further gain.

Both halves of that sentence matter. The brain continues to change, and patients told at twelve months that they have plateaued are frequently told so on the basis of assumption rather than evidence. Meaningful gains years out are well documented. At the same time, some patients do reach a genuine plateau, and for them the healthiest goal is not indefinite pursuit of further recovery but building a life that works within real constraints. A clinician who can only offer the first message will fail the patients who need the second.

The focus in this phase shifts toward sustainability: continued regulation practice, neuroprotective habits around movement, sleep, and nutrition, periodic reassessment, and attention to the identity questions Chapter 10 takes up directly. Many patients in this phase are less troubled by their symptoms than by the question of who they are now, and that question deserves clinical attention rather than referral onward as if it were someone else's domain.

> **Clinician Tip.** Treat this stage as consolidation rather than discharge. Ask whether the patient has sustainable practices they will actually maintain, and whether the goals have shifted from compensation toward capability and meaning. Be careful with "optimization" language: it can imply that continued effort guarantees continued gain, which is not true for everyone and can leave patients feeling that a plateau is a personal failure.
>
> **Teach-Back Tool.** "What is one small way you could include a brain-body practice in your day, even if just five minutes?" The answer tells you more about likely adherence than any plan you construct for them.

CASE EXAMPLE

Marcus, Continued: Gastrointestinal Symptoms Within a Broader Recovery Picture

Marcus's composite story continues here, the same fictional educational composite introduced in Chapter 4, not a real patient.

By the time a year had passed, Marcus's autonomic symptoms had settled into something manageable. What hadn't budged was his cognitive fog and the fatigue that hit him hardest after mentally demanding days, worse than his pacing strategies alone could explain, even though those strategies and his autonomic regulation work had genuinely helped up to that point.

It was only when asked directly that he mentioned the gut symptoms he'd never brought up: irregular digestion, occasional bloating. Nobody treated this as confirmation of anything. It went on the table as a hypothesis to explore alongside his known autonomic pattern, nothing more, and it stayed there deliberately. This case never included mitochondrial or cellular-energy testing, so no claim gets made about that system. A gut-related contributor was simply one more plausible factor worth investigating among several, not a single hidden cause finally found. Whether it was actually contributing anything to his fatigue remained genuinely open.

Before touching anything gut-directed, his pattern got characterized properly: frequency, timing, its relationship to meals and stress, along with his tolerance for dietary change and anything that might contraindicate an approach. Only once there was a real clinical question did specific options come up with him, and even then, with the understanding that not everything suits everyone. Fermented foods, for instance, aren't right for every patient. Whatever changed would need to fit his specific pattern, not arrive as a general bundle handed to anyone with a gut symptom.

Over the following months, Marcus found somewhat greater mental stamina and a more predictable recovery curve after exertion. His fatigue never went away, but it became less severe and easier to plan around. Cognitive fog still showed up on his highest-demand days, and because several changes landed around the same time, there's no way to isolate which one mattered most.

This composite illustrates that persistent GI symptoms alongside a fatigue picture may deserve assessment as part of the whole clinical picture, not dismissal as unrelated to cognition or energy. It doesn't show that gut-directed care resolved his cognitive symptoms, and it can't isolate that intervention as the specific cause of his improvement.

6.4 Enhancing Interdisciplinary Collaboration

ABI recovery requires multiple professionals, and yet real integration remains rare. Conventional and integrative approaches frequently operate in parallel silos, each documenting into a record the other does not read.

Bridging these worlds is difficult, and the difficulty deserves acknowledgment rather than the usual exhortation to communicate better. Many conventional providers are skeptical of PEMF, vagal stimulation, or consciousness-based practice, and **a portion of that skepticism is well founded**. Several of these modalities do have limited ABI-specific evidence, exactly as this book states throughout. A clinician who responds to that skepticism by insisting on the modality has confirmed the skeptic's suspicion. A clinician who responds by agreeing about the evidence, and proposing to track outcomes together, has started a different conversation.

Conversely, integrative providers sometimes lack standardized approaches and documentation habits that make coordination possible. If your notes cannot be read by a neurologist, coordination will not happen regardless of goodwill.

What functional collaboration requires. Shared clinical models that combine functional medicine, neuroscience, and neurorehabilitation around the common targets: metabolic support, neuroimmune regulation, plasticity activation, and autonomic balance. Routine case review, where the whole team evaluates progress and adapts plans rather than each discipline reporting in turn. Cross-disciplinary education, so that a neurologist understands what photobiomodulation is being used for and a speech-language pathologist can recognize autonomic dysregulation when it derails a session.

A shared-case example. A patient with persistent post-concussive symptoms might see a neurologist for diagnostic and pharmacological management, a functional medicine provider for metabolic and gut-brain support, a rehabilitation therapist for cognitive retraining and dual-task integration, and a clinician trained in regulation-based tools. Working independently, these four produce four plans the patient must reconcile alone, usually while cognitively impaired. Coordinating, they produce one plan with sequencing that makes sense: metabolic and sleep work established before cognitive demand escalates, regulation practice timed before rather than after the most taxing sessions, and a single agreed answer when the patient asks what to prioritize this month.

Practical mechanics. Agree on who tracks what, so that HRV data, symptom logs, and functional measures have an owner. Establish explicit handoffs. Tolerate principled disagreement: a physician skeptical of a modality and a therapist enthusiastic about it can coordinate well if both are honest about the evidence and both keep the patient's stated priorities central. What does not work is silent disagreement, where the patient receives contradictory guidance and resolves it by trusting whoever spoke most recently.

> **Action Step.** Establish a regular interdisciplinary check-in to review symptom shifts, refine approaches, and maintain alignment. Weekly is ideal; monthly is far better than never. Consistency matters more than duration.
>
> **Clinician Tip: Scan the Five Bodies.** Train clients to reflect across the Five Bodies (Physical, Vital, Mental, Supramental, Bliss). This gives patients language for experiences that otherwise go unreported, particularly in the domains conventional intake never asks about, and it often surfaces the concern that matters most to them.

6.5 Patient Education and Self-Management

Patient education is central to ABI rehabilitation and structurally difficult, because brain injury impairs precisely the capacities that education depends on. Memory, attention, and executive function are the machinery of learning, and we are asking damaged machinery to absorb complex, unfamiliar, often frightening information.

Verbal instruction and jargon-heavy handouts fail predictably here. Patients nod in the appointment and retain almost nothing by the parking lot, then feel ashamed about it, then disengage. What looks like noncompliance is frequently a comprehension failure that nobody detected.

Effective communication prioritizes accessibility, clarity, and repetition. Multimodal delivery matters: visual aids, simplified step-by-step instructions, written summaries the patient takes home, and demonstration alongside explanation. Reduce the number of things communicated per visit; two remembered points beat six forgotten ones.

The teach-back method is the highest-value tool in this section. Rather than asking whether the patient understood, which reliably produces yes, invite them to restate it: "Can you tell me how you would explain this to someone at home?" This surfaces confusion immediately and lets you correct it while the patient is still in front of you. Done warmly, it does not feel like testing; done as a check on your own clarity rather than their competence, it builds trust.

Caregiver involvement. Family members frequently bridge clinical recommendation and daily implementation, and training them in health literacy extends everything you do. Treat caregivers as co-educators rather than as observers. Also attend to caregiver burden directly, since a depleted caregiver cannot sustain the support the plan assumes.

Education in this model is about capability rather than information transfer. When patients understand why an intervention matters and feel able to carry it out, they become participants rather than recipients, and that shift predicts adherence better than any instructional technique.

> **Teach-Back Tool.** "Can you tell me how you would explain this to someone close to you?" This reinforces learning, surfaces confusion, and builds confidence, and it tells you what actually landed rather than what you said.

6.6 Designing Optimal Healing Environments

Healing happens in environments, and for people recovering from ABI the environment is not background. It is either supporting the nervous system or taxing it, and the difference is clinically consequential.

Conventional clinical spaces frequently tax it. Bright fluorescent lighting, echoing corridors, chemical cleaning odors, and visual clutter overload a system already struggling with sensory processing. Many survivors experience light sensitivity, auditory filtering difficulty, vestibular instability, and heightened environmental reactivity. In these cases the setting itself drives sympathetic activation before the session begins, and the therapy you deliver competes against the room you deliver it in.

Lighting. Natural light supports circadian regulation and mood; soft, indirect lighting reduces overstimulation. Fluorescent lighting with visible flicker is a common and correctable problem. Where overhead lighting cannot be changed, lamps at lower height transform a room cheaply.

Sound. Minimize background noise and provide quiet zones. Attend to constant low-level sources, HVAC hum, electronics, corridor noise, which patients often cannot identify as the problem but respond to when removed. Soft surfaces reduce reverberation inexpensively.

Scent and air quality. Synthetic fragrance and chemical cleaning products are frequent triggers. Fragrance-free policies cost nothing and help a meaningful minority of patients considerably. Ensure ventilation.

Color and visual field. Softer, lower-contrast palettes are generally experienced as calming; busy patterns and high-contrast visual clutter are taxing for patients with visual-processing difficulty.

Temperature and airflow. Thermoregulation is frequently affected after ABI, and patients are often uncomfortable without saying so. Ask.

Beyond sensory input, attend to **psychological safety**: clear visual structure with unobstructed pathways and visible exits, adjustable seating so patients can choose position and distance, predictable routines, and small signals of warmth such as plants or soft textures. These communicate safety nonverbally to a nervous system reading the room before the conversation starts.

Extending this to the home. This is where the leverage is, since patients spend far more time at home than in your clinic. Teach the principles rather than prescribing a setup: a designated low-stimulation space for recovery, consistent evening lighting that dims as night approaches, reduced visual clutter in high-use areas, and attention to the specific triggers that patient has identified. When patients learn to shape their own sensory environment, they gain a real form of agency, and it is one of the few interventions that costs nothing and works immediately.

> **Research Insight.** Sensory features of clinical environments, including light, sound, scent, and spatial layout, influence autonomic function and stress response. For neurologically vulnerable individuals, thoughtful environmental design functions as a therapeutic strategy rather than an amenity. *(Evidence label: environmental and sensory-accommodation recommendations rest on general physiological principles, rehabilitation consensus, and patient-reported outcomes rather than ABI-specific controlled trials. They are low-risk, low-cost, and widely endorsed.)*

6.7 Coaching and Motivational Interviewing

Healing after ABI asks for sustained effort over a long period with unreliable feedback. Patients work hard for weeks and cannot always tell whether it is helping. Under those conditions, motivation is not a personality trait; it is something the clinical relationship either supports or erodes.

Motivational interviewing is a conversational method for strengthening a person's own motivation for change. It rests on empathy, nonjudgment, and the premise that patients are the experts on their own lives. It deliberately avoids confrontation, guiding instead toward the person's own values and resolving ambivalence through curiosity. This suits ABI recovery well, where survivors frequently face overwhelm, fatigue, and a damaged sense of their own competence.

Four techniques carry most of the weight:

Open-ended questions that invite exploration rather than steering. "What matters most to you as you recover?" often produces an answer that reorders the treatment plan. Patients name returning to a specific role, activity, or relationship far more often than they name a functional measure.

Affirmations that recognize specific effort rather than offering generic praise. "You have kept that morning routine going for three weeks, including the weeks it was hard" lands differently from "you're doing great," because it demonstrates that you were paying attention.

Reflective listening that rephrases to confirm understanding and to let the patient hear themselves. "It sounds like you are discouraged, and you have not given up" holds both halves of an ambivalence the patient may not have articulated.

Summarizing that links parts of the conversation and consolidates direction. "So your main goals are managing fatigue and feeling more in control of your day. Let us focus there" converts a diffuse conversation into a plan the patient recognizes as theirs.

Coaching shifts the emphasis toward forward movement: helping patients rebuild agency, reframe identity, set their own milestones, and troubleshoot obstacles. The clinician functions as facilitator rather than fixer, which is a substantial change in posture for many of us and takes practice to sustain when a patient is struggling and the fixing instinct is strong.

Adapting for cognitive and communication impairment. This is where standard MI training frequently falls short, because it assumes conversational capacities many ABI patients do not currently have. Slow the pace considerably. Use short, concrete language. Ask one question at a time and tolerate the silence while it is processed, which will feel longer to you than it is. Offer visual supports: goal boards, simplified checklists, written summaries of what was decided. Invite responses through gesture, drawing, or pointing when speech is effortful. Watch nonverbal cues, which often carry the answer when verbal output is limited.

Autonomy as clinical substance. Trauma-informed care emphasizes choice, and it does so for reasons that are physiological as well as ethical. Patients with ABI have typically experienced a catastrophic loss of control, frequently followed by a medical system that made decisions for them. Restoring genuine choice, even over small things, reverses part of that experience. Offering two options rather than one instruction is a small change with disproportionate effect on engagement. It also produces better plans, because patients choose what they can actually sustain.

A worked example. A patient says they have not been doing their home program. The instinctive response is to restate its importance. The more useful response is curiosity: what got in the way? The answer is frequently structural rather than motivational, the program takes forty minutes they do not have, or requires a quiet room they do not have, or produces symptoms they were not warned about. A program the patient can actually complete, even a reduced one, outperforms an ideal program they cannot.

6.8 Language and Reframing Techniques

Words shape how patients interpret their own experience, and interpretation shapes engagement. In ABI care, where frustration and grief are constant companions, the language a clinician uses is a working tool.

Neuro-Linguistic Programming offers a set of communication strategies for this, and an honest note about it belongs here rather than in a footnote. **NLP as a formal theoretical model has not been empirically validated, and its original neurological claims**

are not supported by evidence. Its practical techniques, however, overlap substantially with well-established cognitive-behavioral and motivational-interviewing methods, and those overlapping practices are what this section recommends. Framed that way, the techniques are useful and honestly presented. Framed as validated neuroscience, they would not be, and clinicians who present them that way to colleagues will lose credibility they need for more defensible parts of this work.

Reframing changes how a person interprets a challenge without denying the challenge. Fatigue understood as the nervous system requesting recovery prompts a different response than fatigue understood as failure. Slow progress understood as consolidation prompts a different response than slow progress understood as a ceiling. These shifts are not cosmetic; they alter the emotional and physiological response to the symptom, and they change what the patient does next.

The practical technique is to listen for the interpretation embedded in what the patient says and offer an alternative that is equally true. When a patient says "I cannot remember anything anymore," the statement is both an observation and a verdict. A response like "your memory is still reorganizing, and you have already built tools that support it" keeps the observation and replaces the verdict.

> **Action Step: Communication techniques for clinical practice.**
>
> - **Pacing and leading.** Meet the patient's current state first ("it sounds like this has been hard"), then extend toward possibility ("and even so, here you are again"). Leading without pacing reads as dismissal.
> - **Sensory language matching.** Notice how the patient describes their experience and respond in kind. Someone who says "I just cannot picture it" may respond to a sketch; someone who says "it doesn't feel right" may respond to a somatic check-in.
> - **Future pacing.** Guide the patient to imagine a specific successful scenario: "What would it look like to get through Thursday with energy left over? What would you notice first?" Specificity matters; vague optimism does little.
> - **Chunking.** Break overwhelming goals into parts small enough to start today. "Let us organize the morning" is actionable in a way "rebuild executive functioning" is not.
> - **Gentle suggestion.** "As you take a breath, you might notice focusing becomes a little easier." Use with discretion, and never in a way the patient would object to if it were explained.

Reframing Phrases Reference

When patients express frustration.

Patient says	Possible reframe
"I am so slow now."	"Your brain is asking you to move more mindfully, and that is okay."
"I cannot do anything right anymore."	"You are learning to do things differently, and that takes strength."
"This is taking forever."	"Healing takes time, and every step is part of the process, including this one."

When patients criticize their cognition.

Patient says	Possible reframe
"My memory is gone."	"Your memory is still reorganizing. Let us work with it rather than against it."
"I keep messing up."	"Mistakes are part of rebuilding. Each one shows you what works."
"I am not the same person."	"You are becoming someone new, with new strengths and insights."

When patients feel overwhelmed by tasks.

Patient says	Possible reframe
"It is too much. I do not know where to start."	"Let us take one small step at a time and build clarity together."
"I keep forgetting everything."	"Your brain is working hard. We can use tools to support it."
"I should be further along by now."	"Progress looks different for everyone. You have already come a long way."

Reframing tips. Mirror their language briefly before offering a new frame. Use "still," "yet," and "becoming" to signal that the situation is in motion. Emphasize progress over perfection. Keep tone unhurried. When uncertain, ask: "What would it feel like to see this differently?"

> **Clinician Tip.** Reframing is not about dismissing real pain, and the distinction matters. Used to hurry a patient past genuine grief or loss, reframing becomes invalidation with a friendly face, and patients recognize it immediately. The test is whether the reframe is also true. "You are becoming someone new" is true and useful; it is not a substitute for letting someone grieve who they were.

> **Teach-Back Tool.** Ask your client or group how they would use breath, sound, or posture to settle their nervous system. Having them demonstrate rather than describe reinforces embodied learning.

6.9 Digital Tools, Data Tracking, and Assistive Technology

Digital tools, self-monitoring, and adaptive aids increasingly shape rehabilitation, and they fit the emphasis on extending care into daily life. This section names specific products where naming them is useful, and it distinguishes carefully among four things that are easy to conflate.

> **How to read the tools below.** For each category, this section separates: **(a)** evidence for the *modality* in general; **(b)** evidence for any *specific product*, which is usually far thinner; **(c)** whether the tool is **clinician-directed** (requiring training, interpretation, or prescription) or a **consumer wellness** tool the patient can adopt independently; and **(d)** cost and availability, which change and should be verified. **Named products are examples of a category, not endorsements.** Evidence that a modality works does not establish that a particular device implementing it works, and this distinction is where most product marketing operates.

Self-tracking and wearables

Modality evidence. HRV is a well-supported marker of autonomic function and is among the most useful repeatable measures in ABI care, given how central autonomic dysregulation is to this population. Sleep and activity tracking support pacing decisions and give patients concrete feedback.

Commonly used tools. The **Oura Ring** and **WHOOP** provide HRV, sleep staging, and readiness metrics with minimal user effort, which suits patients whose executive function makes manual logging difficult. **Apple Watch** and **Fitbit** offer broader health tracking with wide availability and lower cost of entry. **Elite HRV** provides morning HRV readings using a chest strap, which is generally more accurate than wrist or finger optical sensors for beat-to-beat variability.

Product-specific evidence and limits. Consumer device *accuracy varies substantially* by device, sensor type, and context. Chest-strap ECG-based measurement outperforms optical sensors for HRV; sleep staging from consumer wearables correlates only moderately with polysomnography and should not be treated as diagnostic. None of these devices has meaningful ABI-specific outcome evidence. What they offer is consistent, low-burden trend data, and trend within a single device is far more meaningful than absolute values or cross-device comparison.

Category: consumer wellness, clinician-interpreted. **Cost:** subscription models are common and change frequently; several require ongoing payment beyond the hardware. Verify current pricing before recommending, and consider that a subscription is a recurring burden for patients who have lost income.

Biofeedback and neurofeedback devices

Modality evidence. HRV biofeedback has reasonable support for autonomic regulation and anxiety. EEG neurofeedback has a substantial general literature for attention and regulation with important methodological debates and limited ABI-specific outcome data.

Commonly used tools. HeartMath Inner Balance provides real-time HRV coherence training with an accessible interface, widely used in clinical and home settings. The **Muse** headband offers consumer EEG-based meditation feedback. **Apollo Neuro** delivers patterned vibration intended to influence autonomic state. Clinical neurofeedback systems, including **NeurOptimal** and practitioner platforms trained through **EEGInfo**, require certification and clinical oversight.

Product-specific evidence and limits. HeartMath's coherence approach has a reasonable body of supporting work, much of it produced by the affiliated institute, which is worth knowing when weighing it. Consumer EEG headbands use few electrodes and are not equivalent to clinical EEG; they are meditation-support tools rather than assessment devices, and should never be presented to patients as brain measurement in a diagnostic sense. Apollo Neuro's supporting evidence is preliminary. **Clinical neurofeedback is a clinician-directed intervention requiring training and certification**, and qEEG findings alone do not prescribe a protocol.

Category: HeartMath and Muse are consumer wellness; clinical neurofeedback is clinician-directed. **Cost:** consumer devices range from modest to substantial; clinical neurofeedback courses represent a significant patient expense, frequently uncovered.

> **Caution: Overuse of Feedback Devices.** Too much stimulation from PEMF, neurofeedback, or HRV tools can overwhelm sensitive clients. Begin with short sessions and track tolerance. Headache, fatigue, or agitation may signal a need to pause or scale back. More device time is not better, and patients inclined toward effort will need to hear that explicitly.

Cognitive training and symptom-tracking applications

Modality evidence. Computerized cognitive training reliably improves performance on trained tasks. **Transfer to untrained real-world function is much weaker and should not be implied to patients.** Symptom and mood tracking supports pattern recognition and shared decision-making.

Commonly used tools. BrainHQ and **Lumosity** are widely used cognitive training platforms with exportable progress data. **Bearable** tracks symptoms, mood, and lifestyle factors together, which suits the multi-symptom picture typical after ABI. **Daylio** offers low-friction mood and activity logging with minimal typing, useful when writing is effortful. **Reflectly** provides guided journaling. **Tally** tracks simple habits such as hydration or practice adherence.

Product-specific evidence and limits. BrainHQ has more published supporting work than most competitors, including trials in older adults, though transfer claims remain contested and marketing in this sector has been subject to regulatory action historically. Tracking applications are conveniences rather than validated instruments; their value is adherence and pattern visibility, not measurement precision.

Category: consumer wellness. **Cost:** subscription-based, changing frequently, with free tiers of varying usefulness.

Purpose-built recovery applications

Worth knowing specifically because they are **free, evidence-informed, and publicly available**, which makes them among the most practical recommendations in this chapter for cost-constrained patients. The US Department of Veterans Affairs publishes **CBT-i Coach** (structured support for cognitive behavioral therapy for insomnia, the first-line treatment for chronic insomnia), **PTSD Coach**, **Concussion Coach**, and **Mindfulness Coach**. **Insight Timer** offers a large free library of guided practice. **10% Happier** and **Peak** are subscription alternatives in mindfulness and cognitive training respectively.

A note on CBT-i Coach specifically: because CBT-I has strong evidence and poor availability, a free structured application supporting it addresses a real access gap. It works best alongside clinician guidance rather than alone.

Category: consumer wellness, several developed by public health agencies. **Cost:** free for the VA applications and Insight Timer's core library.

External cognitive supports

Modality evidence. External memory aids have among the **strongest rehabilitation evidence** of anything in this section, particularly for moderate-to-severe injury. This is well established and frequently underused.

Memory books are personalized binders or journals holding key facts, photographs, routines, contacts, and therapy tasks. Build them with the patient during sessions, using their own language and images, since ownership drives use. **Health passports** provide a portable summary of diagnoses, medications, preferences, and communication needs, valuable during care transitions and urgent visits and particularly for patients with aphasia or cognitive-communication difficulty. **Orientation aids** including large-print calendars, visual timers, labeled photo directories, and "today is" boards anchor time and place and reduce the anxiety of disorientation.

Low-technology versions often outperform applications here, because they require no login, no charging, and no navigation.

Category: clinician-directed in design, patient-owned in use. **Cost:** minimal.

Augmentative and alternative communication

Modality evidence. AAC is well established for expressive and receptive communication impairment, and should also be considered for patients with cognitive fatigue or situational communication barriers rather than reserved for severe aphasia alone.

Commonly used tools. Low-technology AAC includes communication boards, picture and topic cards, and dry-erase templates. High-technology options include **Proloquo4Text** and **Proloquo2Go**, **Grid 3**, and **Lingraphica** devices, several of which are designed specifically for acquired communication disorders and may be fundable through insurance as durable medical equipment.

Product-specific note. AAC selection should be made **with a qualified speech-language pathologist** through formal assessment, not chosen from a list. Fit depends on motor access, vision, literacy, cognitive profile, and context of use, and a poorly matched device is typically abandoned. Funding pathways differ substantially by device and payer, which is itself a reason to involve an SLP who knows them.

Category: clinician-directed. **Cost:** ranges from negligible to several thousand dollars; insurance coverage is often available for dedicated devices with appropriate documentation.

Integration in practice

A patient with autonomic dysfunction might track HRV each morning, log symptoms in a simple application, and time demanding activity around energy patterns. A memory book might hold their therapy summary, exercise photographs, and weekly reflections. A health passport might streamline an emergency visit. An AAC tool might allow participation in group therapy while speech recovers.

The unifying principle is that each tool should answer a question that changes what you or the patient do. Tools that generate data nobody acts on generate burden.

Teaching Data Literacy

Self-tracking only helps when patients can interpret what they are seeing. Without guidance, patients misread normal fluctuation as deterioration, chase numbers, or develop anxiety about metrics that were meant to reassure them.

This risk is real and worth naming. For patients prone to health anxiety, perfectionism, or rumination, daily biometric tracking can become another arena for self-criticism. For those patients, less tracking is the better clinical decision, and saying so explicitly relieves them of the sense that they are failing at yet another thing.

Teach patients to watch **trends rather than points**. A single low HRV reading means little; noticing that HRV improves after a restful evening and drops after a demanding day is actionable. Use simple visuals to support pattern recognition, and pair device data with subjective notes, since the correlation between what the device says and how the patient feels is itself informative and sometimes surprising.

Reassure patients that improvement is rarely linear. Most usefully, help them connect data to decisions: if Tuesday's numbers predict a hard Wednesday, what changes on Tuesday evening? That question turns tracking into agency rather than surveillance.

6.10 Overcoming Barriers to Adoption

Integrating this model into mainstream practice is hard. Healthcare systems resist change, clinicians are overburdened, administrators are risk-averse, and reimbursement rarely accommodates emerging approaches. These barriers are real, and a chapter that treated them as attitude problems would be useless.

Clinician hesitancy. Many professionals were never trained in these approaches and reasonably regard some as unproven. The productive response is to engage the skepticism rather than to overcome it rhetorically. Lead with the interventions that have the strongest evidence and the lowest barrier: sleep, pacing, HRV biofeedback, graded activity, nutrition. These are defensible in any setting and give a skeptical colleague something to agree with. Track outcomes and share them, including the disappointing ones, because a colleague who sees you report a negative result will trust your positive ones.

> **A caution on imaging as persuasion.** The original chapter suggested using SPECT and qEEG imaging to demonstrate improvement and win clinician buy-in. This warrants care.

> Current VA/DoD guidance advises against routine use of neuroimaging, including functional imaging, to establish post-acute mTBI diagnosis or to direct treatment, and neither SPECT nor qEEG findings by themselves demonstrate clinical improvement. Using images persuasively, when they cannot support the inference being drawn, undermines exactly the credibility this section is trying to build, and a colleague who knows the guidance will notice.

Institutional resistance. Hospitals and rehabilitation centers operate under insurance-driven efficiency models with little tolerance for unbillable time. Some interventions map onto existing rehabilitation categories; documentation matters here, and framing regulation work in functional terms it actually serves is both accurate and practical. Partnering with academic institutions can enable grant-funded pilots that generate data while limiting financial exposure. Claims about cost savings should be framed as hypotheses to test locally rather than as established findings, because administrators have heard confident savings claims before.

Patient engagement. Many survivors are unfamiliar with these approaches and are already managing more appointments than they can track. Simplicity wins. Framing a specific, small, achievable trial, "let us try five minutes of this and see whether your afternoons change," builds more trust than a comprehensive plan that overwhelms on presentation.

Financial and accessibility barriers. This deserves more weight than it usually receives. Patients with ABI frequently lose income precisely when expenses rise, and an enthusiastic clinician can do real harm by recommending a stack of devices, supplements, and testing that a family cannot afford but will attempt anyway. Begin with what costs nothing: sleep, light timing, pacing, breathwork, hydration, movement, education, environmental modification. These carry much of the available benefit. Add cost only where the added value is clear, and say out loud that the free interventions are not the lesser ones. **A version of this care that costs a patient nothing should always be available, and should be offered first.**

Geographic and access barriers. Trained practitioners cluster in metropolitan areas. Telehealth addresses part of this, and much of the highest-value work, education, pacing, sleep, coaching, regulation practice, translates well to remote delivery. Where local specialists are unavailable, clinicians can often supervise foundational work themselves rather than referring indefinitely.

6.11 Implementation Timeline and Team Roles

A structured rollout helps, and the sequence matters more than the calendar. Assemble the clinical team and define roles. Train staff on initial approaches. Run a pilot with a selected patient group while monitoring adherence and outcomes. Adjust based on what the pilot reveals, which will not be what you predicted. Then move to fuller implementation with continued evaluation. A roughly sixteen-week arc suits many settings; a smaller practice may move faster, and a hospital system will move slower.

The pilot phase is the one most often skipped and the one that matters most, because it produces local evidence and surfaces workflow problems while they are still cheap to fix.

Roles. Neurologists provide medical oversight and neurological assessment. Nutrition professionals develop dietary approaches. Occupational, physical, and speech-language therapists lead functional and neuroplasticity work. Psychologists provide emotional and cognitive-behavioral support and hold the trauma-informed frame. Nurses or care coordinators track adherence, manage scheduling, and maintain communication, a role frequently underestimated and frequently the reason programs hold together or fall apart.

Meeting structure. Useful prompts sound like: "Given this patient's assessment findings, should we adjust the approach?" or "Based on these results, what should we prioritize this month?" Rotate who presents, so the meeting does not become a series of parallel reports.

Action area	Guiding approach	Considerations
Program rollout	Phased: team setup, training, pilot, full implementation	Build in review checkpoints; expect the pilot to change the plan
Interdisciplinary collaboration	Regular structured team meetings on shared cases	Documentation should promote clarity and shared responsibility
Patient education and literacy	Teach-back, simplified explanation, visual aids	Confirm understanding each visit; adapt to cognitive and emotional readiness
Adherence barriers	Structured routines and consistent follow-up	Flex plans to energy, rhythms, and patient-reported obstacles
Integrative technology	HRV tracking first, then others where trained and indicated	Begin with no-cost regulation tools; ensure trauma-informed integration
Nervous-system feedback	HRV or wearable data for regulation trends	Keep monitoring sustainable; avoid data overload

> **Mind-Body Reflection: Your Nervous System Sets the Tone.** Before each session, check in with yourself. Are you regulated or rushing? Present or distracted? Your own state becomes part of the container for your client's work, and patients with ABI are unusually sensitive to it. How might you reset in small ways between appointments?

6.12 Frequently Asked Questions

Q: What supplements support neurometabolic healing after brain injury? Nutrients including CoQ10, NAD+ precursors, omega-3 fatty acids, and alpha-lipoic acid are commonly used to support mitochondrial function and reduce oxidative load. Decisions should follow clinical findings, symptom patterns, and interaction checking rather than protocol. Evidence for most of these in ABI specifically is mechanistic rather than outcome-based, and cost is a legitimate clinical consideration. Where a patient can afford either supplements or nutritious food, food is the better recommendation.

Q: Is there an ideal frequency or protocol for PEMF in ABI care? No, and it is worth saying so plainly rather than implying that one exists somewhere in the literature. Device type, waveform, intensity, and tolerance vary widely, and the evidence base does not support a standard setting. PEMF should be used by trained practitioners, introduced conservatively, and guided by response. Be skeptical of any source presenting a universal protocol.

Q: How can diet and lifestyle influence gut-brain healing? Anti-inflammatory, whole-food approaches including prebiotic fiber, fermented foods, and gut-supportive nutrients may support microbiome diversity and reduce inflammatory load. The gut-brain axis also responds to stress regulation, so vagal support, mindfulness, and hydration belong in the same conversation. Benefits for ABI recovery specifically remain plausible rather than established.

Q: How often should dual-task training or mental rehearsal be used? Frequency should match capacity and phase. Some patients tolerate daily engagement; others need shorter, spaced sessions. The useful question is not how often but how well matched the practice is to current readiness. If a session reliably produces a two-day recovery cost, the dose is wrong regardless of what the schedule says.

Q: What about detoxification protocols? Supporting the body's own clearance through sleep, hydration, movement, fiber, and nutrition is reasonable and low-risk. Aggressive commercial detoxification protocols, and chelation outside documented heavy-metal toxicity, are not supported for ABI recovery and carry genuine risk in a population already prone to fatigue and sensitivity. The distinction between supporting physiology and purchasing a protocol is worth making explicit with patients, who encounter a great deal of marketing in this space.

Q: How do I talk about interventions whose evidence is limited without either overselling or dismissing them? Say what you know. "This has good evidence for X, less for your situation specifically, and here is what I would watch for" is a sentence patients respond well to. Uncertainty stated plainly builds more trust than confidence that later proves unfounded, and it models the reasoning you want patients to apply to the marketing they will encounter without you.

Chapter 6 Quick-Reference Guide and Summary

Core concepts.

- **Four program layers:** neurometabolic optimization, neuroplasticity-driven rehabilitation, bioelectromagnetic regulation, consciousness and relationship-centered healing, sequenced because lower layers enable upper ones.
- **Three recovery phases:** stabilize (0 to 3 months), train with precision (3 to 12 months), consolidate and sustain (12 months and beyond), with honest acknowledgment that plateau is real for some patients.
- **Interdisciplinary collaboration:** shared targets, routine case review, cross-disciplinary education, and skepticism engaged rather than dismissed.
- **Patient education:** multimodal, teach-back-verified, caregiver-inclusive, and limited to what can actually be retained.
- **Healing environments:** light, sound, scent, color, temperature, and psychological safety as clinical variables, extended into the home where the leverage is greatest.
- **Coaching and MI:** open questions, affirmations, reflective listening, summarizing, adapted for cognitive and communication impairment, with autonomy as clinical substance.
- **Language and reframing:** useful communication practice, presented honestly as overlapping with CBT and MI rather than as validated neuroscience, and never used to hurry someone past grief.
- **Digital and assistive tools:** named examples with modality evidence, product evidence, clinician-directed versus consumer status, and cost distinguished throughout; external memory aids and AAC carry the strongest support.
- **Barriers:** clinician hesitancy, institutional constraint, patient engagement, cost, and geography, each with practical responses, and a no-cost version of care always available.

Practical clinical actions.

- Start with the highest-evidence, lowest-cost, lowest-disruption interventions and prove them locally.
- Match intensity to measured readiness rather than to elapsed time since injury.

- Verify understanding every visit rather than assuming it.
- Introduce technology only where it answers a question that changes management, and scale back when it overwhelms.
- Offer the free version of this care first, and mean it.

Chapter 7: Holistic Symptom Management in ABI

Multisystem, bioelectromagnetic, and integrative approaches

7.1 The Case for Multisystem Healing

ABI presents with a range of symptoms that rarely resolve when treated in isolation. Fatigue, brain fog, mood instability, chronic pain, gastrointestinal difficulty, hormonal shifts, and sleep disturbance often coexist, reflecting disruption across neurological, endocrine, immune, and autonomic systems.

Conventional care tends to fragment these complaints: a medication for sleep, a referral for memory, a supplement for energy, each addressed by a different provider who sees one facet. Patients cycle through this and frequently report that nothing helped much, which is a reasonable conclusion when each intervention addressed one node of a network without touching the network.

Viewing symptoms as signals of dysregulation, whether neuroinflammation, mitochondrial impairment, autonomic imbalance, or the physiological residue of trauma, lets us address contributing drivers rather than only managing discomfort. This is not a claim that everything is connected in some vague sense. It is a specific clinical observation: after ABI, poor sleep worsens inflammation, inflammation worsens fatigue and mood, fatigue drives inactivity, inactivity worsens autonomic function and sleep, and the loop closes. Interrupt it at any point and several symptoms move together. This is why patients sometimes report that fixing their sleep improved their headaches, their digestion, and their temper simultaneously, and why chasing each of those separately so often fails.

An honest framing note. The interventions in this chapter span a wide evidence range, from well supported (sleep and circadian work, CBT-I, graded activity and pacing, vestibular rehabilitation, pituitary screening) through reasonable and low-risk (botanical support, breathwork, environmental modification) to frankly investigational (frequency-based tools for specific symptoms). This chapter labels them as it goes. The goal is not symptom suppression but restoration of regulation, pursued honestly.

How to prioritize. When a patient presents with eight symptoms, treating all eight is neither possible nor wise. Ask which one, if it improved, would most improve the others. That is usually sleep. Then ask which is most treatable and most commonly missed, which points toward the screening list in §7.16. Start there rather than with the symptom the patient finds most distressing, while explaining why, because a patient whose headaches are the worst part of their week deserves to know why you are asking about their breathing at night.

ABI Symptom Matrix

Symptom cluster	System affected	Primary intervention targets
Brain fog, fatigue	Mitochondrial, clearance pathways, sleep	Sleep optimization, pacing, metabolic support, graded activity
Anxiety, panic	Autonomic, vagal, limbic	Breathwork, HRV biofeedback, vagal toning, adaptogens, mental health referral
Headaches, pressure	Neurovascular, cervical, medication effects	Hydration, magnesium, cervical assessment, medication-overuse screening
Constipation, bloating	Gut-brain axis, vagal, dietary	Fiber, gut repair, vagal support, red-flag screening
Poor sleep, irritability	Limbic and circadian, sleep-disordered breathing	Apnea screening, CBT-I, light timing, wind-down routine
Low motivation, apathy	Dopaminergic tone, mood, isolation	Depression screening, behavioral activation, movement, light, social contact

> **Note on the matrix.** This grid supports pattern recognition; it does not prescribe. A symptom cluster can have several drivers, and low motivation in particular should prompt screening for depression rather than being treated only as a neurochemical or supplement question. Appendix C provides the fuller navigation matrix with system categories and chapter cross-references.
>
> **Mind-Body Reflection: Your Rhythm Becomes the Model.** Are your clinical habits reinforcing the rhythms you want clients to embody? Where do your daily patterns reflect regulation, and where might they invite recalibration? Patients notice whether we live what we recommend, and the ones who are paying closest attention are often the ones struggling most.

7.2 Cognitive Dysfunction: Brain Fog and Processing

Cognitive complaints are among the most common and distressing post-ABI symptoms: difficulty concentrating, mental fatigue, slowed processing, and word-finding trouble. Patients describe reading a paragraph four times, losing a thought mid-sentence, or finding conversation exhausting in a way it never was.

These difficulties are often rooted not in structural damage alone but in multiple contributors: neuroinflammation, impaired energy metabolism, poor sleep, autonomic dysregulation, medication effects, and mood. This matters clinically because the contributors are addressable in ways that structural damage is not, and because patients who believe their fog is permanent structural loss behave differently from those who understand it as a state with modifiable inputs.

Conventional cognitive rehabilitation has genuine evidence (Cicerone et al., 2019) and belongs at the center of care. Integrative work complements rather than replaces it, addressing the physiological conditions that determine whether cognitive rehabilitation can take hold. A patient sleeping five fragmented hours will not consolidate what they practice, however well the practice is designed.

Sleep is frequently the highest-yield intervention here and is regularly underweighted. Before adding cognitive supplements, ask about sleep quality, apnea symptoms, and sleep timing. The gain from correcting a sleep problem typically exceeds anything else available for fog.

Practical approaches. Address sleep and circadian rhythm first (§7.12). Support metabolic capacity through nutrition and blood-sugar stability. Reduce inflammatory load where drivers are identified. Use pacing so that cognitive work happens in the window where the patient has capacity, which for many is mid-morning. Teach cognitive strategies and external supports rather than relying on effort alone. Address mood, since depression produces cognitive symptoms indistinguishable from injury-related ones and is treatable.

> **Research Insight: Adaptogens.** Adaptogenic botanicals including *Rhodiola rosea*, *Withania somnifera* (Ashwagandha), *Bacopa monnieri*, and *Ginkgo biloba* have been studied for effects on stress response, cognitive performance, and neuroprotection. *(Evidence label: most trials are in non-ABI populations, healthy adults or general stress and anxiety, with small samples and heterogeneous preparations. Verified examples include Chandrasekhar, Kapoor, & Anishetty (2012) for Ashwagandha and Olsson, von Scheele, & Panossian (2009) for Rhodiola, both in non-ABI populations. These are reasonable adjuncts with real interaction potential, not established ABI treatments, and they should be introduced after foundational work rather than instead of it.)*
>
> **Caution: Botanical Interactions.** Adaptogens are pharmacologically active. Check interactions before recommending, particularly with anticoagulants, thyroid medication, sedatives, immunosuppressants, and antihypertensives. Ashwagandha specifically warrants caution in thyroid disease, pregnancy, and autoimmune conditions, and has case reports of hepatotoxicity. Ginkgo affects bleeding risk. Start low, introduce one agent at a time so that effects and adverse reactions are attributable, and coordinate with prescribing clinicians.

7.3 Fatigue: Rebuilding Energy and Resilience

Fatigue after ABI is often profound, persistent, and misunderstood by everyone around the patient. Unlike ordinary tiredness it is systemic and rest-resistant; patients describe a heaviness that makes a shower feel like a decision. Families frequently interpret it as depression or lack of effort, and patients often internalize that interpretation.

It reflects neurological strain along with HPA-axis dysregulation, disrupted diurnal rhythm, mitochondrial demand, autonomic imbalance, and the enormous cognitive cost of doing consciously what used to be automatic. Many describe a "tired but wired" state: exhausted yet unable to settle, which points toward autonomic rather than simply energetic depletion.

Pacing is the foundational intervention and has better support than any supplement in this section. The typical pattern is boom-and-bust: patients feel adequate, do everything they have been postponing, crash for two days, then repeat. Each crash costs more than the good day gained. Structured activity management, taking rest *before* fatigue rather than in response to it, breaks this cycle and often produces more functional gain than any addition to the regimen.

Teaching pacing well takes more than telling patients to rest. It requires helping them identify their actual tolerance, plan around it, and tolerate the emotional difficulty of stopping while they still feel capable, which many experience as giving up. Framing pacing as the thing that expands capacity over time, rather than as accepting limitation, is usually necessary for adherence.

Graded aerobic activity, introduced carefully and titrated to tolerance, is included in guideline recommendations for persistent post-concussion symptoms, although the recommendations are weak and based on low to very low certainty evidence (Rytter et al., 2021). It remains among the better-evidenced active interventions available, which says as much about the state of the field as about the intervention. The titration matters; too much too soon reproduces the crash cycle with clinical endorsement attached.

Foundational supports matter more than supplementation: consistent wake time, morning light, adequate protein, hydration with attention to electrolytes, and blood-sugar stability across the day. Adaptogens are commonly used as adjuncts, with Rhodiola sometimes used for daytime energy and Ashwagandha or Holy Basil for evening hyperarousal, subject to the interaction cautions above.

Screen for the treatable contributors that masquerade as post-injury fatigue: sleep apnea, anemia, thyroid dysfunction, post-traumatic hypopituitarism (§7.8), depression, and medication effects. Several are common, all are treatable, and each is regularly attributed to the injury and left alone for years.

Clinician Tip: Anchor Habits to Existing Routines. New practices stick better when attached to something already happening. Pair morning light with the first cup of coffee; pair breathwork with a commute or the school run. Executive-function demand is the main barrier to adherence in this population, so reduce it. A practice that requires remembering, deciding, and initiating will fail; one attached to an existing cue often survives.

7.4 Pain and Central Sensitization

Pain after ABI frequently does not correspond to imaging findings, or occurs without structural damage at all. These presentations are not imaginary; they reflect disrupted neural feedback, central sensitization, and altered pain processing. Neuroinflammation and impaired descending inhibition contribute to a state in which ordinary input is interpreted as threatening.

Chronic pain in this context becomes less about tissue damage and more about the nervous system's interpretation of internal state. This is a useful clinical insight and also one that must be communicated carefully, because "your nervous system is interpreting" sounds to many patients like "it is in your head," which is precisely what they have been told dismissively by others.

Pain neuroscience education has good support and is often the highest-value first step. Teaching patients how sensitization works, that pain is produced by the nervous system's threat appraisal rather than measuring tissue damage directly, changes the appraisal that drives it. Patients frequently report that understanding this reduces both fear and pain. It works because it is true and because it relieves the interpretation that every flare signals new damage.

Graded activity and movement follow. Avoidance maintains sensitization; graded exposure reduces it. The pacing principles above apply.

Somatic awareness. Many patients hold chronic protective contraction in the jaw, diaphragm, shoulders, or pelvic floor without awareness. Gentle micro-movements, body scanning, and somatic tracking invite the nervous system out of bracing. These are low-risk and often produce noticeable relief in a single session, which builds confidence in the broader approach.

Adjunctive supports. Photobiomodulation and PEMF are sometimes used for local inflammation and sensory regulation at an investigational level. Topical and botanical supports including magnesium, arnica, and capsaicin-based preparations may modulate pain signaling. Nervine herbs such as skullcap and passionflower are used for evening flares that disrupt sleep.

Emotional pain and somatic expression. Grief, anger, fear, and unprocessed trauma frequently express through the body, and naming this possibility, as an integrated feature of human experience rather than as pathology, can allow patients to approach pain with curiosity. Name it carefully and late rather than early. Patients with ABI have usually already been told their symptoms are psychological, and a clumsy version of this observation repeats that harm and ends the therapeutic relationship. Earn the standing to raise it, and raise it as a possibility alongside the physiological work rather than as a replacement for it.

7.5 Headaches

Post-traumatic headache is common and almost always multifactorial. Cervical contributors, vascular components, medication overuse, sleep disruption, dehydration, visual and vestibular strain, and autonomic instability interact, creating feedback loops of discomfort and fatigue.

A systems approach outperforms symptomatic suppression. **Cervical and suboccipital assessment matters**, since cervicogenic contributors are frequently missed when the presentation is attributed entirely to the brain injury. Manual approaches including suboccipital release are used clinically; craniosacral therapy carries limited evidence and is best framed as comfort-oriented rather than corrective.

Magnesium is a reasonable, inexpensive, well-tolerated first-line supplement here, with better support in headache than in most applications in this book. **Anti-inflammatory botanicals** including feverfew, turmeric, and boswellia are used, with feverfew having the more developed migraine-prevention literature.

Medication-overuse headache deserves explicit screening. It is common, treatable, easily missed when everything is attributed to the injury, and actively worsened by the analgesic use it drives. Ask specifically how many days per week the patient takes something for headache. The answer frequently surprises both of you.

Visual and vestibular contributors should be assessed (§7.6), since visual strain is a common headache driver in this population and responds to intervention.

Environmental and lifestyle factors. Light sensitivity and screen aggravation are frequent. Screen dimming, glare reduction, adjusted font size, and scheduled visual breaks help. **A caution on tinted lenses:** routine indoor use can worsen photophobia over time through adaptation, so tinted wear should be purposeful and time-limited rather than continuous. Sleep regularity and blood-sugar stability play meaningful roles, and protein-containing breakfasts, avoiding caffeine on an empty stomach, and regular meals prevent the dips that trigger headaches in many patients.

Frequency-based tools applied to occipital or frontal regions are used at an investigational level, best combined with breathwork or HRV work that addresses autonomic contributors.

Above all, patients need validation. Persistent headaches are not weakness or exaggeration. Reframing them as feedback about cumulative load, rather than as failure, helps patients respond with adjustment instead of frustration.

> **Clinician Tip: Assess Hydration.** Dehydration is a common and easily corrected headache contributor here, particularly in patients whose fatigue reduces fluid intake, whose autonomic symptoms have led them to restrict, or who have simply stopped noticing thirst. Ask what they actually drank yesterday rather than whether they drink enough.

7.6 Vision and Vestibular Dysfunction

Vision and vestibular problems are among the most underrecognized yet disruptive consequences of ABI. Patients report dizziness, spatial disorientation, nausea, photophobia, or visual strain, often struggling to describe what is wrong. They say they feel "off," avoid grocery stores and busy environments, or cannot read for more than a few minutes. These complaints are frequently dismissed or attributed to anxiety when they reflect genuine sensory integration problems.

After injury, coordination among ocular tracking, visual-vestibular integration, and proprioception can be impaired. Even modest deficits such as convergence insufficiency or impaired saccades produce substantial cognitive fatigue, because stabilizing vision and navigating space consumes attentional resources continuously. Patients experience this as fog rather than as a visual problem, which is why it goes unidentified.

Early referral to a neuro-optometrist or vestibular-trained physical therapist is the key clinical move, and vestibular rehabilitation has genuine evidence in this population (Galeno et al., 2022). This is among the better-supported interventions in the entire book and should not be buried among adjuncts. Patients who have been unwell for months sometimes improve substantially within weeks of appropriate vestibular or visual rehabilitation, and the delay is usually diagnostic rather than therapeutic.

Screening questions that identify candidates: "Do your symptoms worsen when reading, scrolling, or in visually busy places like supermarkets?" "Does moving your head quickly change how you feel?" "Do you avoid particular environments because of how they make you feel?" Positive answers warrant referral rather than accommodation alone.

While awaiting formal evaluation, clinicians can support recalibration with gaze stabilization exercises, gentle head-turn drills within tolerance, and breathwork. Somatic grounding such as pressing feet into the floor or using weighted lap pads provides proprioceptive input that helps anchor patients who feel unmoored. Introduce these gradually; provocation is common and should guide dosing rather than being pushed through.

Adjuncts. Magnesium and ginger are sometimes used for vestibular excitability and nausea, ginger having reasonable antiemetic support. Screen filters, glare reduction, and adjusted display settings help visual strain.

Practical tool. The 20-20-20 approach: every 20 minutes of visual work, look about 20 feet away for roughly 20 seconds. Simple, free, well tolerated, and easy to remember, which matters in this population.

7.7 Autonomic Dysregulation

Chronic fatigue, light sensitivity, orthostatic dizziness, temperature dysregulation, and emotional volatility may stem from dysautonomia rather than from stress or deconditioning alone (Mercier et al., 2022). Chapter 4 develops assessment; this section addresses management.

The clinical picture varies. Some patients are locked in sympathetic dominance: wired, hyperreactive, unable to settle. Others present with parasympathetic collapse: flat, exhausted, lightheaded. Most fluctuate unpredictably between them, which is exhausting in itself and frequently misread as emotional instability.

Breath regulation is the cornerstone and the highest-value starting point. Coherent breathing at roughly five to six breaths per minute supports HRV and vagal tone, and patients often notice a shift within minutes, which makes it excellent for demonstrating that physiological self-regulation is possible (Jerath et al., 2006; Lu et al., 2023 for HRV biofeedback). That demonstration matters beyond its direct effect: a patient who has felt at the mercy of their body experiences something they can influence.

Hydration and electrolytes, particularly adequate sodium, support blood volume and vascular tone, which matters considerably for orthostatic intolerance and is often the single most effective intervention for it.

Graded, position-tolerant exercise, beginning recumbent or seated where standing is poorly tolerated, is an established component of orthostatic intolerance management. Compression garments help some patients.

> **Caution: Dizziness During Breathwork.** If a client becomes dizzy during breathing exercises, particularly with rapid breathing techniques or breath holds, stop. Return to slow diaphragmatic breathing. Assess hydration, blood sugar, and autonomic status. **Avoid hyperventilatory techniques in this population**, including rapid-breathing practices popular in wellness settings; they can provoke significant symptoms in patients with autonomic instability.

Botanical supports including Ashwagandha, Rhodiola, and Holy Basil are used to buffer sympathetic overactivation. **Licorice root requires specific caution**: it raises blood pressure through mineralocorticoid effects and can cause hypokalemia and hypertension. It is sometimes used deliberately in hypotensive patients, and that use requires clinical oversight and monitoring rather than casual recommendation.

PEMF applied to the cervical region or solar plexus is used to shift autonomic tone at an investigational level, often alongside grounding, gentle somatic work, or restorative practices such as yoga nidra.

Validation is a clinical intervention here, not a courtesy. Many patients have been dismissed or told their symptoms are just anxiety, sometimes for years. A physiological explanation is itself regulating, because it converts an experience that felt like personal failure into a condition with mechanisms. Language matters: framing dysautonomia as a state of overwhelm rather than a defect helps shift patients from self-blame toward collaboration.

7.8 Hormonal and Metabolic Dysfunction

Hormonal and metabolic disruption is among the most underrecognized consequences of ABI. Patients experience persistent fatigue, weight change, low libido, mood instability, or thermoregulatory difficulty, frequently dismissed as unrelated, psychological, or simply part of recovery.

The connection is well established. **The pituitary is vulnerable to injury even in mild TBI, and post-traumatic hypopituitarism is a documented phenomenon** (Tan et al., 2017; British Neurotrauma Group guidance). This is one of the strongest evidence-based reasons in this book to look beyond the obvious, and one of the most consequential things in this chapter to miss, because the deficiencies are treatable and the symptoms are often attributed to the injury indefinitely.

Damage can impair signaling across HPA, thyroid, gonadal, and growth-hormone axes. Patients may present with low morning energy and poor stress tolerance, features suggesting thyroid involvement despite results within reference range, or menstrual irregularity, reduced libido, and emotional flattening.

Screening for post-traumatic hypopituitarism should follow published guidance and involve endocrinology where indicated. This is a medical evaluation, not a functional-testing exercise, and framing it correctly matters: a patient sent for expensive functional panels when they need a formal pituitary workup has been poorly served.

From an integrative perspective, the aim beyond deficiency detection is restoring rhythm across systems: sleep and circadian regularity, adequate nutrition, blood-sugar stability, stress load management, and appropriate activity. Some functional testing approaches, including salivary cortisol patterns and dried urine hormone panels, are used clinically but carry **significant validation limitations** and should not substitute for appropriate endocrine workup where deficiency is suspected. Adaptogens support stress-response resilience as adjuncts. Nutrients including B-complex vitamins, magnesium, and vitamin D serve as cofactors, with vitamin D worth actually measuring rather than assuming.

> **Simple intervention: a food and symptom awareness journal.** Track meals and timing, energy before and after eating, mood and focus, sleep quality, movement, and digestive symptoms. Keep it low-pressure; consistency matters more than completeness. Review two or three days together in session to identify correlations, such as an afternoon crash following a skipped breakfast, which patients rarely spot alone. **Where a patient shows preoccupation with food, restriction, or distress about eating, pause this tool** and address the concern directly rather than reinforcing it; detailed food tracking is contraindicated where disordered eating is present or emerging.

7.9 Mitochondrial Support and Cellular Energy

Mitochondrial function is frequently impaired after ABI (Hiebert et al., 2015), contributing to brain fog, fatigue, poor stress tolerance, and reduced capacity for the demanding work of rehabilitation. This is the physiological substrate beneath much of what patients describe as running on empty.

Practical daily supports carry most of the benefit and cost nothing. Morning light exposure within the first hour of waking supports circadian alignment, which in turn supports mitochondrial rhythm. Meals emphasizing adequate protein, healthy fats, polyphenol-rich foods, and micronutrient cofactors provide substrate. Gentle movement, walking, stretching, breath-led yoga, supports mitochondrial biogenesis without triggering crashes, which matters enormously here given post-exertional worsening. Sleep does more for cellular energy than any supplement.

Photobiomodulation is used where accessible, targeting mitochondrial cytochrome c oxidase, at the evidence level described in Chapters 2 through 4.

Supplemental mitochondrial cofactors commonly used include CoQ10 or ubiquinol, NAD+ precursors, alpha-lipoic acid, and acetyl-L-carnitine. *(Evidence label: these rest largely on mechanistic rationale and non-ABI populations rather than ABI outcome trials. They are reasonable and generally well tolerated. Frame them to patients as supportive rather than curative, and weigh cost seriously: a monthly supplement expense that competes with groceries is not a neutral recommendation, and the foundational interventions above outperform them.)*

7.10 Gut Health and Digestive Symptoms

Gastrointestinal symptoms are common after ABI and interact with everything else. Discomfort disrupts sleep, restriction affects nutrition, altered motility affects medication absorption, and vagal involvement links gut and autonomic function bidirectionally.

Approaches include mucosal support with demulcent botanicals such as marshmallow root or slippery elm, zinc carnosine, and glutamine; microbiome support through fiber, fermented foods, and strain-appropriate probiotics; and vagal support to address motility. Introduce gradually, since this population is frequently sensitive and a too-fast introduction produces symptoms that end the trial prematurely.

Practical sequencing. Fiber and fermented foods before supplements. One change at a time so effects are attributable. Attention to eating rhythm and to the autonomic state during meals, since eating in a sympathetic-dominant state impairs digestion regardless of what is eaten.

> **Red flags warranting medical workup rather than integrative management:** unexplained weight loss, bleeding, persistent vomiting, difficulty swallowing, nocturnal symptoms that wake the patient, or new severe pain. These require evaluation before any dietary or supplement approach.

Chapter 6's evidence label applies here too: gut-supportive care is reasonable and low-risk, not proven ABI treatment. The gut-brain axis is well-established biology; that microbiome-directed treatment improves ABI recovery specifically is not established.

7.11 Detoxification and Environmental Sensitivity

Detoxification is often misunderstood, either overemphasized through aggressive commercial protocols or ignored entirely. Both extremes fail patients.

Injury can affect clearance capacity through oxidative load, lymphatic stagnation, altered hepatic function, and reduced physical activity. Concurrent inflammation may increase sensitivity to environmental triggers. Many patients describe a persistent sense of feeling "off" or "sensitive to everything," and that experience is real and worth addressing.

This is not a time for intense cleansing. Interventions should respect limited reserves and proceed gently. Aggressive protocols in a depleted patient produce symptoms, expense, and discouragement.

Foundational support is where the benefit lies: adequate hydration, electrolyte balance, daily movement to support lymphatic flow, fiber and regular elimination, sleep for glymphatic clearance, and nervous-system regulation to reduce overall physiological load. Liver-supportive botanicals such as milk thistle and dandelion may be introduced, with NAC or glutathione support where appropriate.

> **Important safety qualification.** Binders including activated charcoal, chlorella, and zeolite are widely used in integrative practice but have **limited evidence for the indications commonly claimed** and carry real risks: charcoal binds medications and nutrients and must be separated from them by hours, and product quality varies considerably. **Chelation therapy is appropriate only for documented heavy-metal toxicity, under medical supervision, and is genuinely dangerous when used speculatively**, with deaths reported. "Mold illness" and multiple chemical sensitivity remain contested diagnostic areas: the symptoms are real, the diagnostic frameworks and much of the testing marketed alongside them are not well validated, and the associated protocols are frequently expensive. Address confirmed exposures properly and support foundational physiology; avoid committing fatigued, financially stretched patients to speculative programs.

7.12 Sleep and Circadian Rhythm

Sleep disturbance is among the most pervasive symptoms after ABI and among the most consequential. Patients describe fragmented sleep, difficulty falling or staying asleep, non-restorative rest, or early waking, patterns reflecting disrupted neuroendocrine signaling rather than simple insomnia. Injury can affect melatonin and cortisol regulation, limbic circuitry, and arousal pathways, compounded by pain, trauma, hormonal shifts, and environmental overstimulation.

Sleep is a neuroregenerative event rather than merely rest. Without adequate slow-wave and REM sleep, glymphatic clearance is impaired, memory consolidation falters, and repair is compromised. Poor sleep degrades every other domain of recovery, which is why **this is often the single highest-yield target in the entire chapter** and why it deserves attention before most of what precedes it.

Screen for sleep apnea. Sleep-disordered breathing is common after brain injury, frequently missed, and specifically treatable. It should be ruled out before persistent sleep disruption is managed with botanicals and sleep hygiene alone. Patients with unrefreshing sleep, morning headache, witnessed apneas, or resistant fatigue warrant referral. Treating apnea sometimes resolves what looked like intractable post-injury fatigue and fog.

CBT-I is first-line for chronic insomnia, has strong evidence including adapted delivery for cognitive impairment (Edinger & Carney, 2015), and belongs ahead of supplements. Access is the practical barrier; the free CBT-i Coach application (§6.9) partially addresses it.

Circadian entrainment provides the foundation. Natural light within thirty minutes of waking, ideally outdoors, since indoor light is dramatically dimmer than patients assume. Consistent wake time, which anchors rhythm more effectively than consistent bedtime. Protein-containing morning meals. Daytime movement. Evenings reverse this: dimmed lighting, reduced screen exposure, and a wind-down routine that reliably signals downshift.

Supportive measures include warm baths, topical magnesium, calming herbal teas such as passionflower, chamomile, or lemon balm, and slow breathing. **Melatonin** has reasonable evidence for circadian rhythm disruption specifically, at lower doses than commonly sold, and is better suited to timing problems than to sleep-maintenance insomnia; dosing and timing matter more than quantity.

The psychological dimension. Anxiety about sleep perpetuates sleeplessness, and by the time patients reach us many have been fighting their sleep for months. Addressing that loop, through CBT-I principles including stimulus control and reducing time-in-bed, is frequently more effective than adding another sleep aid to a growing collection.

7.13 Hearing and Auditory Processing

Hearing difficulties after ABI are common and frequently overlooked, affecting communication, cognitive processing, fatigue, and social participation. Patients may hear normally on an audiogram and still be unable to follow conversation in a restaurant.

Auditory processing evaluation comes first. Comprehensive audiometric testing and auditory processing assessment identify difficulty understanding speech in noise, sound hypersensitivity, tinnitus, and auditory fatigue. Referral to audiology is the appropriate step rather than presumptive management.

Sound therapy and auditory retraining use white or pink noise and calibrated approaches with graded exposure to reduce hypersensitivity. **Graded exposure has support in hyperacusis management, and complete sound avoidance tends to worsen sensitivity over time.** This point deserves explicit conversation with patients seeking silence for relief, since the intuitive response makes the problem worse and patients need to understand why we are asking them to do something uncomfortable.

Neuroplasticity-driven auditory rehabilitation engages targeted auditory tasks, dual-task work combining auditory with visual or motor demand, and rhythmic auditory stimulation, which has reasonable support in gait and timing applications.

Nutritional support including omega-3s, antioxidants, zinc, and magnesium is used for cochlear health at a mechanistic rather than established evidence level.

Tinnitus specifically has better-supported management through sound therapy and CBT-based approaches than through supplementation, and patients should be told this directly rather than cycling through supplements that will not help. Tinnitus distress responds to treatment even when the tinnitus itself persists, which is a hopeful message worth delivering.

Practical accommodations matter: preferential seating, reduced background noise during appointments, written summaries, and permission to use noise-reducing headphones in taxing environments, with the caution above about avoidance.

7.14 Environmental Exposures and EMF

Neurotoxic exposures, including heavy metals, pesticides, and mold, can affect neurological function, and documented exposure warrants proper medical evaluation and remediation. Assessment involves appropriate testing interpreted by qualified clinicians. **Hair mineral analysis and many direct-to-consumer toxin panels have poor validity and frequently generate expensive, anxiety-driven interventions on the basis of unreliable results**, which is a substantial practical problem in this patient population.

Regarding electromagnetic fields, honesty is required. Patients sometimes report headaches, sleep disturbance, and cognitive symptoms they attribute to EMF exposure from routers, phones, and other devices. Blinded provocation studies have not demonstrated that individuals can detect EMF exposure under controlled conditions, and current evidence does not support non-thermal EMF exposure at typical environmental levels as a cause of these symptoms.

The symptoms are entirely real and often severe. The attribution is what remains unsupported. Holding both halves of that sentence is the clinical task.

This distinction can be handled with compassion and to the patient's benefit. Reducing device use in the evening does help sleep, through light exposure, cognitive stimulation, and timing rather than through field effects. Recommending that change is reasonable and effective. Recommending shielding products, EMF meters, or home remediation is not supported and can be actively harmful: it entrenches an explanatory model that isolates patients, drains resources they need, and can escalate into avoidance that shrinks their world.

Where a patient holds this attribution strongly, arguing rarely helps and often ruptures the relationship. The clinical priority is to stay engaged, treat the real symptoms effectively, and avoid actively reinforcing the model. Patients whose symptoms improve through sleep, pacing, and autonomic work frequently revise the attribution themselves.

7.15 Patient and Practitioner Perspectives on Symptom Management

Two perspectives are worth naming here, because symptom management is where they most often collide.

From the patient's side, the dominant experience is of accumulating explanations that did not fit. Most have been told their fatigue is depression, their dizziness is anxiety, their fog is stress, and their pain is deconditioning. Some of these were partly true. All of them, delivered without curiosity, taught the patient that describing their symptoms produces dismissal. By the time they reach an integrative clinician, many are braced for it, and some present their history defensively or with more certainty than the evidence supports because they have learned that tentativeness invites dismissal.

From the practitioner's side, this creates a genuine tension. You will sometimes disagree with a patient's explanatory model, as in the EMF discussion above. Handling that without either capitulating or dismissing is the skill this chapter most requires. What works is to validate the experience completely and unconditionally, be honest about the explanation when asked, and let effective treatment do the persuading over time.

The convergence: take the symptoms entirely seriously, hold the explanations lightly, and stay in the relationship long enough for the physiology to answer the question.

CASE EXAMPLE

Theo: Safety, Co-Regulation, and Engagement with Care

The following is a fictional educational composite representing a commonly seen pattern in trauma-informed brain injury care, not a real patient.

By the time Theo reached this clinic, he'd already cycled through several providers. He was two years out from a severe brain injury, and the pattern with him was consistent: missed appointments, sessions where he seemed to shut down and stop participating. Earlier care had focused on cognitive and physical rehabilitation goals, reasonably enough, but with little attention paid to how unsafe or dismissed Theo had felt in healthcare settings before this one. He clearly cared about his own recovery when he did show up. So why the inconsistency? There wasn't an obvious single answer.

Before reaching for the explanation that felt easiest, that this was about safety and trust, the team checked the practical ground first. Prospective-memory difficulty that made him forget appointments rather than avoid them. Executive-function challenges with planning and follow-through. Transportation, caregiver support, fatigue relative to when his sessions were scheduled, whether he could actually follow what was being communicated during a visit, financial and logistical strain. Several of these turned out to be real and relevant. And alongside them, Theo talked about specific past experiences in healthcare that had felt dismissive or unpredictable.

Both mattered, and treating this as only a logistics problem or only a trust problem would have missed half of what was actually happening. So the response addressed the concrete barriers directly, reminder systems, caregiver coordination, sessions timed around his fatigue pattern, while also changing how care itself was delivered: predictable structure, real choices, a clinician presence that stayed calm and consistent. No new biomedical intervention entered the picture during this phase. That wasn't the point yet.

What shifted was Theo's attendance, steadier now, and the way he talked about his own symptoms, in more detail, with less minimizing. He started taking a more active role in decisions about his own care. His underlying cognitive and physical symptoms didn't change through any of this; they remained their own separate, ongoing piece of work.

What this composite illustrates is that inconsistent engagement after brain injury is often both a practical problem and a safety problem at once, and that addressing them together, rather than picking one, is what actually moved things. What it doesn't show is that co-regulation or trauma-informed practice resolved Theo's neurologic symptoms, or that relational care is a substitute for biomedical treatment.

7.16 Bringing It Together

Symptoms after ABI are not fixed defects but expressions of a system attempting to rebalance. Fatigue, fog, mood changes, pain, digestive distress, and sleep disruption are layered signals of dysregulation. Interpreted through a systems lens they cohere as interconnected narratives rather than unrelated complaints, which is what allows a small number of well-chosen interventions to move several symptoms at once.

What this population needs is not more protocols. They need context, and clinicians who can connect symptoms, systems, and interventions, who will pause, listen, and build plans matching their physiology, capacity, and actual life.

The screening list worth running on everyone, because each item is common, treatable, and regularly missed: sleep-disordered breathing; medication-overuse headache; post-traumatic hypopituitarism; vestibular and visual dysfunction; depression and anxiety; medication side effects; thyroid dysfunction and anemia; and nutritional inadequacy. Finding one of these changes a patient's trajectory more than any addition to their supplement regimen.

The Symptom Management Matrix enhances clinical reasoning rather than replacing it. Healing is not linear, and patients benefit most when care is layered, individualized, and responsive to what changes.

Chapter 7 Quick-Reference Guide and Summary

Core concepts.

- **Multisystem framing.** Symptoms as interacting signals of dysregulation, which is why targeted intervention moves several at once.
- **Highest-yield targets:** sleep (apnea screening, CBT-I, circadian entrainment), pacing, vestibular and visual referral, pituitary screening, hydration and electrolytes. These carry the strongest evidence and belong first.
- **Reasonable adjuncts:** botanicals with interaction checking, breath and somatic regulation, environmental modification, mitochondrial support.
- **Investigational:** frequency-based tools for specific symptom domains.
- **Explicitly qualified:** binders and chelation, functional hormone panels, direct-to-consumer toxin testing, EMF attribution.

Practical clinical actions.

- Run the screening list for the treatable and commonly missed before elaborating the regimen.

- Lead with sleep, pacing, light timing, hydration, and graded activity; add cost only where value is clear.
- Check botanical interactions every time and introduce one agent at a time.
- Teach pacing as capacity-building rather than as limitation, or it will not be followed.
- Validate symptoms unconditionally while remaining honest about which explanations the evidence supports.

Chapter 8: Future Directions in ABI Care

Rehabilitation is entering a period of change. Tools that were speculative a decade ago are in trials; tools that were in trials are in clinics. For a clinician trying to serve patients well, this creates an uncomfortable position: dismissing everything new fails patients who might benefit, and adopting everything new fails patients who pay for things that do not work.

The discomfort is not a problem to be solved. It is the correct response to an honest situation, and clinicians who feel it are usually paying attention. What follows is not a way to eliminate that tension but a way to hold it usefully.

This chapter maps that territory. Per the author's decision, emerging, translational, technological, and consciousness-based material is **restored in full and calibrated through evidence labels rather than removed**. Forward-looking work belongs in a clinician's guide, because clinicians are asked about it by patients who have already found it online and want to know what to think. A patient who arrives with a printout about focused ultrasound has not made an error. They have done what any reasonable person does when conventional care has not fully answered their situation. The clinician who has never heard of the technology, or who dismisses it reflexively, loses standing in that conversation and often loses the patient's willingness to raise the next question.

What that requires is honesty about status. The most useful thing this chapter can give you is not a verdict on each technology but a habit of asking the right question: not "does this work?" but "what exactly is being claimed, what evidence supports that specific claim, and in whom?"

A posture to name. There is a stance available here that is neither credulous nor dismissive, and it is harder to hold than either. Credulity is comfortable because it lets you offer hope without qualification. Dismissal is comfortable because it protects you from being wrong in public. The demanding position is sustained curiosity inside firm boundaries: genuine interest in what might become possible, combined with an unwillingness to present possibility as fact. This posture is not a compromise between the other two. It is a discipline, and it asks something specific of clinicians, which is the tolerance to say "I find this interesting and I do not yet know" without experiencing that as failure.

Four questions to carry through this chapter. Applied to any emerging intervention, these do most of the evaluative work:

10. **What is it actually doing?** Not what it is marketed as doing. What is the proposed physical or physiological mechanism, stated plainly enough that its claims can be checked?
11. **What clinical question would it answer?** Every technology should map to a problem clinicians recognize. If it does not solve a problem you have, its novelty is not relevant to your patients.
12. **What evidence exists, in whom?** Mechanistic plausibility, animal work, healthy-volunteer studies, adjacent clinical populations, and ABI-specific trials are five different things that are frequently discussed as if they were one.
13. **What would responsible adoption require?** If you cannot describe the conditions under which you would use it, you do not yet understand it well enough to offer it.

> **How to read this chapter.** Every section carries a status label:
>
> - **Available now** with reasonable evidence.
> - **In trials**, with early or mixed human data.
> - **Preclinical or theoretical**: promising mechanism, no human outcome data.
> - **Speculative**: worth tracking, not supported by current evidence.
>
> Nothing here should be offered to patients as established care on the strength of this chapter alone.

8.1 A Necessary Correction on Sourcing

There is a lesson in that correction beyond the numbers themselves, and it applies to reading this literature generally. A precise figure feels like evidence. It carries the texture of measurement, and it is easy to repeat. But a percentage is only as good as the study behind it, and in emerging fields the studies behind circulating percentages are frequently small, uncontrolled, unpublished, or absent altogether. When a striking number cannot be traced to a specific paper with a specific population and a specific outcome measure, the appropriate clinical response is not to discount the topic. It is to discount the number and go looking for what is actually known.

8.2 Artificial Intelligence in Neurorehabilitation

Status: in trials, with some components available now.

What it is. In rehabilitation contexts, artificial intelligence generally refers to algorithmic systems that take in streams of data, performance scores, EEG signals, heart rate variability, movement kinematics, and adjust the parameters of a task in response. The term covers a wide span, from simple adaptive difficulty rules that a spreadsheet could implement, to machine-learning models trained on large clinical datasets. That span matters, because "AI-powered" on a product page tells you almost nothing about which of these is inside.

The clinical question it might answer. Conventional rehabilitation follows parameters a clinician adjusts periodically, usually between sessions and based on observation. The problem this creates is one every clinician recognizes: the patient who was appropriately challenged at the start of a session is overwhelmed by minute twenty, and the session's second half produces frustration rather than learning. Algorithmic systems can analyze performance and physiological signals continuously and adjust within the session, aiming to keep the patient at the edge of their capacity rather than above or below it.

Why this matters conceptually. The optimal challenge point is a real phenomenon: too easy produces no adaptation, too hard produces failure and disengagement, and that point moves within a single session as fatigue accumulates. This is not a minor scheduling detail in ABI. Fatigue in this population is not ordinary tiredness but a physiological ceiling that arrives quickly and shifts day to day, and working above it does not simply produce less learning. It can produce symptom exacerbation that costs the patient the following day as well. Human therapists track this well and cannot track it continuously across every parameter. This is the opportunity, and it is worth understanding as an amplification of clinical attention rather than a replacement for it.

Adaptive neurofeedback is the leading example. Traditional protocols set success thresholds adjusted occasionally by the clinician. Adaptive systems monitor EEG continuously, detect changes in state or learning rate, and adjust in real time. The rationale is sound and the technology exists. What remains limited is high-quality controlled evidence that adaptive systems outperform well-delivered standard protocols in ABI populations specifically. That is a meaningful gap, not a fatal one. It is also a familiar shape of gap: the comparison that matters is rarely against no treatment, and a technology can be better than nothing while being no better than the competent conventional care it is priced above.

Wearable integration and remote delivery address a real access problem. Home-based EEG and HRV devices make consistent practice feasible for patients whose fatigue, transport limitations, or geography make frequent visits impractical. For rural patients and those who cannot drive after injury, this is not a convenience but the difference between receiving care and not. That deserves a moment, because access is frequently treated as a secondary consideration in discussions of new technology when it is often the primary one. A moderately effective intervention a patient can actually receive will outperform a superior intervention they cannot reach.

What remains unknown. Whether within-session adaptation produces better functional outcomes than skilled between-session adjustment in ABI. Whether gains transfer beyond the trained task, which is the recurring weakness of computerized cognitive training generally. How long benefits persist after the system is withdrawn. And whether the physiological signals these systems read, particularly consumer-grade EEG and optical HRV, are precise enough to justify the decisions being made from them.

Honest limits, stated plainly. AI tools inherit the limitations and biases of their training data, and rehabilitation datasets underrepresent many populations. Algorithmic recommendations require clinical oversight rather than deference, particularly when a system's confidence exceeds its evidence. Consumer-grade EEG is not clinical-grade measurement and should never be presented to patients as brain assessment. And data privacy deserves more attention than it receives: neurological and physiological data collected by consumer devices is often covered by terms permitting broad use and onward sharing. A clinician recommending a device should be able to answer where the patient's data goes, and most of us currently cannot.

The ethical questions underneath. Three deserve more attention than they usually receive. The first is opacity: when a system recommends a parameter change and cannot explain why, the clinician is asked to defer to reasoning they cannot inspect, which sits awkwardly with professional responsibility for the outcome. The second is consent: patients agreeing to adaptive systems are frequently consenting to continuous physiological monitoring without understanding the scope of what is collected or where it goes. The third is quieter and slower, which is the possibility of clinical deskilling. If the system tracks fatigue, the clinician may stop tracking fatigue, and the skill that made the clinician valuable in the first place erodes through disuse. None of these are reasons to avoid the technology. They are reasons to adopt it deliberately rather than by default.

What responsible adoption would require. Validation in ABI populations rather than extrapolation from healthy volunteers or other diagnoses. Transparency about what the system measures and how it decides. A clinician override that is expected rather than exceptional. Clear data governance the clinician can explain to the patient in plain language. And a cost that is defensible against the alternative uses of the same money.

Practical guidance. Where an adaptive system is available and affordable, it is reasonable to use as an adjunct with realistic framing. Where it is expensive, the burden of proof is higher, because the comparison is not against nothing but against well-delivered conventional care plus the other things that money could buy.

8.3 Virtual and Augmented Reality Rehabilitation

Status: available now, with growing evidence.

What it is. VR-based rehabilitation places the patient in a computer-generated environment, usually through a headset, where tasks can be constructed, graded, and measured. Augmented reality overlays digital elements onto the real environment rather than replacing it, which matters for balance and mobility work where seeing the actual floor is not optional.

The clinical question it might answer. Rehabilitation has a long-standing ecological validity problem: performance in a quiet therapy room with a supportive clinician frequently fails to predict performance in a supermarket. Patients who complete clinic tasks competently return home and cannot manage a kitchen. VR allows graded, repeatable, ecologically meaningful practice: a virtual kitchen requiring sequencing and executive function, a navigation task, a balance environment with controlled visual flow. Difficulty scales to performance, and the system records precise data on what the patient actually did.

Genuine advantages. Engagement, which matters more than it sounds in a population facing months of repetitive practice. Precise control of difficulty and of specific variables such as visual flow or distractor load. Objective performance data. Safe practice of tasks that would be risky in reality, such as street crossing or cooking. And the ability to grade exposure for patients whose difficulty is environmental complexity itself.

That last point matters, because it is the one least well served by conventional rehabilitation. For many patients with ABI, the disabling problem is not any single impaired function but the accumulation of sensory and cognitive demand in ordinary settings. A supermarket is not hard because of any one of its features. It is hard because of light, sound, movement, decision-making, and time pressure arriving together. Conventional therapy has no reliable way to deliver that combination at a tolerable dose and build upward. A controllable environment does, and this is a legitimate reason for clinical interest independent of any technological enthusiasm.

Evidence. Reasonably developed in stroke rehabilitation; ABI-specific evidence is growing but thinner. The mechanism is not mysterious, it is task-specific practice with better control, which is why the evidence has developed relatively quickly.

What remains unknown. Whether gains in virtual environments transfer to the real environments they simulate, which is the central question and remains incompletely answered. What dose is appropriate. Whether AR outperforms VR for mobility and balance work, as its design would suggest. And whether the engagement advantage persists past novelty, which is a question about months rather than sessions.

Practical constraints that matter in this population. VR provokes vestibular symptoms, visual strain, and cybersickness, precisely the symptoms many ABI patients already have. This is not a minor caveat; it is the main reason VR fails in ABI settings. Screen for visual and vestibular dysfunction first, introduce short exposures, and titrate. Patients with convergence insufficiency or vestibular hypersensitivity may tolerate very little initially and considerably more after vestibular rehabilitation, so a poor early trial does not necessarily mean the tool is wrong for them, only that the sequence was.

That sequencing point generalizes well beyond VR, and it is one of the more useful ideas in this chapter. A tool that fails when introduced at the wrong moment is frequently recorded in the chart as a tool that failed. The distinction between "this does not work for this patient" and "this did not work at this point in this patient's recovery" is clinically substantial and easily lost.

What responsible adoption would require. A vestibular and visual screen before first exposure. Short initial sessions with explicit stop criteria the patient controls. A plan for what the virtual practice is meant to transfer to, since practice without a transfer target is entertainment. And attention to whether the patient can afford the equipment if home practice is part of the plan.

8.4 Transcranial Ultrasound Stimulation

Status: in trials, early.

What it is. Transcranial ultrasound stimulation uses focused ultrasonic waves through the skull to modulate specific brain regions. It is mechanical rather than electrical, which distinguishes it from the more familiar non-invasive techniques. Its clinically distinguishing feature is depth: unlike TMS and tDCS, which principally affect cortical surface, TUS can reach structures such as thalamus and hippocampus, which are frequently relevant to ABI-related cognitive, memory, and arousal difficulty.

The clinical question it might answer. A significant portion of persistent post-ABI difficulty appears to involve deep and subcortical structures and their networks: arousal regulation, attention gating, memory consolidation, autonomic control. Existing non-invasive neuromodulation cannot reach most of these directly. If depth were achievable non-invasively and safely, it would open a category of target that is currently addressable only indirectly or surgically. That is a substantial clinical question, and it is why the technique attracts serious research attention rather than only enthusiasm.

What the research shows. Low-intensity TUS has demonstrated capacity to modulate neural activity and, in animal work, to induce long-term potentiation, the cellular process underlying learning. Experimental application to peri-infarct tissue in stroke has been associated with changes in inflammation and connectivity. Ultrasound-based approaches to vagal stimulation are being explored as a non-implanted route to autonomic modulation, which would be clinically significant if it holds.

The disorders-of-consciousness work. The original chapter described a European trial applying focused ultrasound to the thalamus in patients with severe TBI and disorders of consciousness, with a previously unresponsive patient beginning to follow commands. Work of this kind exists and is interesting; thalamic modulation is a rational target given the thalamus's role in arousal and consciousness.

Why caution is essential here specifically. Spontaneous fluctuation in disorders of consciousness is common, recovery trajectories are variable, and single dramatic responses frequently fail to replicate. This is also the patient population where families are most desperate and most vulnerable to overinterpretation. A clinician discussing TUS with such a family carries real responsibility to convey both the promise and the current absence of established benefit. TUS is an area to watch closely, not to offer.

The ethical weight of this particular conversation. Of everything in this chapter, this is the topic where a clinician's words carry the most consequence, and it is worth preparing for rather than improvising. Families of patients with disorders of consciousness are frequently making decisions about continued treatment, and they are doing so exhausted, grieving, and searching. Into that situation, a report of a single patient following commands after thalamic stimulation lands with enormous force. The clinician's task is neither to remove hope nor to inflate it, and there is a real difference between "this is being studied and I will tell you what I learn" and "this might be what your daughter needs." The first respects both the science and the family. The second borrows credibility the evidence has not earned, and when it does not come true, the family absorbs a second loss on top of the first.

What remains unknown. Nearly everything that would be needed for clinical use: which parameters produce which effects, appropriate dosing and spacing, durability of any effect, safety across repeated exposure, which patients might respond, and whether effects observed in group data translate to individual benefit.

What responsible adoption would require. Participation in properly approved research rather than clinical provision. Referral pathways to legitimate trials for interested patients. And clear communication that trial participation is not treatment, which patients and families frequently conflate.

8.5 Advanced Electromagnetic and Resonance Devices

Status: mixed. PEMF is emerging; "quantum resonance" devices are speculative.

Development continues in PEMF, including lower-intensity protocols aiming at deeper targeting and algorithmically optimized parameter selection based on individual response. This is a reasonable extension of the existing evidence discussed in Chapters 2 through 4, and the direction of travel, more individualized parameters rather than fixed protocols, matches what the evidence suggests.

That direction is itself informative. The absence of a universal PEMF protocol has often been read as a weakness of the evidence, and in one sense it is. But it may also reflect something true about the biology: if response depends on individual physiology, injury pattern, and current state, then the search for one correct protocol was misconceived from the start, and parameter individualization is the appropriate scientific response rather than an evasion. This does not make current devices more validated than they are. It does suggest what a mature version of this field would look like, which is a useful thing to know when evaluating claims that the field has already arrived there.

A distinction that matters commercially and clinically. Devices marketed as "quantum resonance" scanners or therapies, which claim to scan the body's frequencies and deliver corrective ones, **are not supported by evidence, and several such products have been subject to regulatory action for unsupported claims.** These are frequently expensive and marketed directly to patients with chronic conditions, including brain injury. Clinicians will encounter patients who have purchased them, and the useful response is neither endorsement nor ridicule but a straight answer about what is and is not established.

How to have that conversation. This situation arises often enough to prepare for. A patient who has spent significant money on an unvalidated device is not in a neutral position, and neither ridicule nor silent agreement serves them. Ridicule tends to produce defensiveness and the loss of future disclosure, which means the next purchase happens without your knowledge. Silent agreement is a form of endorsement. What tends to work is separating the experience from the explanation: the patient's report of feeling better is data about them and is not in dispute, while the device's account of why is a separate claim that the evidence does not support. That separation allows the clinician to be honest without calling the patient foolish, and it keeps open the more important question of what the patient is seeking that conventional care has not provided. Frequently the answer is agency, or attention, or hope, and those are addressable within legitimate care.

The original chapter's vision of future "frequency prescriptions," specifying particular devices and durations by day of week, is retained here as **speculative vision** rather than clinical guidance. It is a reasonable picture of where enthusiasts expect the field to go, and it is not a description of validated practice.

The original also suggested collaborating with energy healers as part of building a future team. That is a matter of individual practice philosophy and patient preference. What this book can say is that any such collaboration should be adjunctive, transparent to the patient, clearly labeled as to its evidence status, and never a substitute for indicated medical care.

> **Mind-Body Reflection: Energetic Hygiene.** What do you absorb from clients: anxiety, grief, urgency? Do you have a way to reset after emotionally intense sessions? Reflect on your boundaries: where do they serve connection, and where might they need tending? Whatever framework you hold about this, the underlying clinical fact is well established, clinicians who do not attend to their own regulation burn out, and burnout degrades care.

8.6 Biofield Measurement Technologies

Status: speculative.

The original chapter proposed combining gas-discharge visualization analysis with HRV biofeedback, EEG, and metabolic testing to build personalized plans from "real-time energetic biomarkers."

Honesty requires separating these components rather than presenting them as a suite. HRV, EEG, and metabolic testing are real measurements with known properties, known limitations, and established interpretation. **GDV and similar biofield imaging technologies have not been validated as measures of a biofield.** Their outputs are substantially influenced by skin moisture, contact pressure, temperature, and ambient humidity, which is a straightforward physical explanation for readings that appear to change with a person's state.

What would validation actually require? This question has a full answer, because the answer is a transferable skill rather than a verdict on one device. A measurement earns clinical use by demonstrating four properties. It must be **reliable**, producing consistent results on repeat measurement of an unchanged subject and across different operators. It must be **valid**, corresponding to the thing it claims to measure rather than to something else, which is precisely where skin moisture and contact pressure defeat the biofield claim. It must be **specific**, distinguishing the target state from other states rather than moving with any change in arousal or hydration. And it must be **responsive** in a way that informs decisions, meaning that a change in the reading should reliably indicate a change worth acting on.

Applied to GDV, the failure is at the second property and it is not marginal. When a known physical confounder fully accounts for the observed variation, the measurement has not been shown to measure the proposed construct at all. Applied elsewhere, the same four questions do useful work: they explain why HRV is clinically usable despite being imperfect, why consumer EEG should not be presented as brain assessment, and why some functional laboratory panels carry the limitations described in Chapter 4 and Appendix D.

These should not be presented to patients as diagnostic imaging, used to justify treatment decisions, or billed as assessment. The concept is retained here as part of the field's exploratory territory, clearly labeled, because clinicians should be able to recognize and discuss it when patients ask.

There is a further reason for a clinician to understand this well rather than simply avoid it. Patients are shown these images, and the images are persuasive in a way that numbers are not. A colorful representation of a person's energy field, presented alongside a practitioner's interpretation, produces conviction. Undoing that conviction later, particularly when treatment decisions have been built on it, is considerably harder than being present with a clear explanation the first time the patient raises it.

8.7 Consciousness-Based Approaches

Status: mixed. Expectancy effects are well established; non-local claims are not.

This section covers the widest evidence range in the chapter, from among the best-established phenomena in clinical medicine to among the least supported, which is exactly why the distinctions matter. The range is also instructive in itself. "Consciousness-based" is not an evidence category. It is a grouping by theme, and grouping by theme is how well-supported practices come to be dismissed alongside unsupported ones, and how unsupported claims come to borrow credibility from their better-evidenced neighbors. Disaggregating such categories is a habit worth developing.

Expectation and placebo effects are real, measurable, and clinically usable. Expectation modulates pain perception, engages endogenous opioid and dopaminergic systems, and influences functional outcomes across conditions. This is not a curiosity at the margins of medicine; it is a substantial and reproducible effect that operates alongside every intervention we deliver.

The clinical implication is larger than it first appears. If expectancy operates alongside every intervention, then it is never a question of whether expectancy is present in a session but only of what it has been shaped toward. The clinician who says "most people find this difficult at first" and the clinician who says "let us see what you can do with this" have both engaged expectancy, and neither has been neutral. Recognizing this does not license manipulation. It removes the illusion that saying nothing was a neutral option.

Clinicians can engage it ethically by maintaining a hopeful, encouraging environment, framing interventions positively where honestly warranted, marking real gains explicitly, and communicating confidence in the patient's capacity. None of this requires deception, and all of it is good practice independently.

> **An ethical boundary worth stating plainly.** It is sometimes suggested that therapists may use "pretend biofeedback," showing a patient a rising bar as though it reflected their brain activity, to produce improvement. **This is deception and should not be practiced.** It is incompatible with informed consent, it destroys the therapeutic relationship when discovered, and it contradicts the same paragraph's own statement that the takeaway is not to use deception.
>
> **Open-label placebo** is the ethical alternative and has a real, growing evidence base: patients are told directly that they are receiving an inert or expectancy-based intervention, told why it may still help, and frequently benefit anyway. This is a striking finding that deserves to be better known, because it means clinicians do not have to choose between honesty and harnessing expectancy. It also fits this population well, since patients who have been dismissed are unusually sensitive to being managed rather than informed.

The deeper principle underneath that correction should be stated directly, because it recurs throughout integrative practice. Any technique that requires the patient not to understand what is happening carries a hidden cost that is usually paid later, and in ABI it is paid with interest. These are patients who have frequently been disbelieved by prior clinicians, told their symptoms were psychological, or managed rather than informed. Discovering that a trusted clinician was also managing them does not simply end one intervention. It confirms a conclusion many of them already suspected, which is that clinicians cannot be trusted with the truth about their own condition, and that conclusion is expensive to reverse.

Meditation, visualization, and intention practices have reasonable support for stress regulation, attention, and wellbeing, and are low-risk and meaningful for many patients. Claims that focused intention directly repairs neural tissue exceed the evidence. The demonstrable effects run through attention, stress physiology, engagement, sleep, and expectancy, which is a substantial enough set of mechanisms that overclaiming is unnecessary.

That last observation generalizes. A recurring pattern in this field is that a practice with solid, well-understood mechanisms gets promoted using a speculative mechanism instead, and the speculative claim then becomes the reason skeptical colleagues dismiss the practice entirely.

The patient loses access to something that would have helped, on the strength of a claim that was never needed to justify it.

Non-local healing and remote intention represent the most contested area. Studies of distant prayer and remote intention have produced inconsistent results, with better-controlled trials generally showing no effect. The original chapter's guidance, to remain open but skeptical and to permit family prayer or distant-healing practices as complementary rather than substitutive, is reasonable and is retained. Families who find meaning in these practices are drawing on real sources of support and community, and there is no clinical reason to interfere.

There is a distinction here that keeps clinicians on solid ground. Permitting, supporting, and not interfering with a family's meaning-making practices is different from making clinical claims on their behalf. A clinician can say without hesitation that a family's prayer is welcome in the room and that their presence appears to settle the patient. The same clinician should not say that the prayer is producing neurological recovery. The first is hospitality and accurate observation. The second is a claim the evidence does not support, and it is not needed for the family to be welcomed.

The accompanying case example, in which a team observed physiological stabilization during family sessions with a comatose relative, is retained with its original caveat that this may reflect the calming environment, familiar voices, coincidence, or the family's own regulation. Familiar voices and reduced ambient stress have plausible physiological effects that require no non-local mechanism.

Biophoton emission research is retained as a theoretical thread. Cells do emit ultra-weak photons; claims that mental states meaningfully alter this emission in ways relevant to healing are speculative and not established.

8.8 Psychedelic-Assisted Approaches

Status: in trials for psychiatric indications; not established for ABI.

Research into psilocybin, MDMA, and related compounds has produced meaningful results in psychiatric conditions, with MDMA-assisted therapy studied for PTSD and psilocybin for treatment-resistant depression. Mechanistically, these compounds are associated with increased BDNF and dendritic spine density in preclinical work, which is why they attract interest for neuroregeneration specifically rather than only for mood.

Why ABI clinicians are interested. Two distinct possibilities, worth separating because they have different evidence and different plausibility. The first is biological: whether a period of heightened plasticity could be paired with rehabilitation to improve motor or cognitive outcomes. The second is psychological: whether these compounds could help patients process the trauma of injury, address the grief and existential distress that follow catastrophic change, or reduce the psychological barriers that keep some patients from engaging in rehabilitation at all. The second is closer to the demonstrated psychiatric evidence and is arguably the more realistic near-term application.

The distinction matters, because the two hypotheses would require different trials, different outcome measures, and different safety frameworks. A study pairing a plasticity window with intensive motor training is a rehabilitation trial. A study addressing post-injury grief and identity disruption is a psychotherapy trial in a medically complex population. Conflating them, which happens frequently in enthusiastic writing, produces the impression of a larger evidence base than exists for either.

What is honest to say. Preclinical plasticity evidence is real (Ly et al., 2018). Human trials in psychiatric populations are meaningful and increasingly rigorous. **There are no established human ABI trials supporting these compounds for brain-injury recovery.** Microdosing specifically has weaker evidence than supervised full-dose protocols, with several placebo-controlled studies finding effects largely attributable to expectancy, which is itself an interesting finding given §8.7.

Safety and legal considerations belong in the body of this section rather than as a footnote. These substances remain controlled in most jurisdictions, and the regulatory picture is shifting unevenly. In ABI populations specifically there are added concerns: seizure risk, psychiatric vulnerability including psychosis risk, medication interactions particularly with serotonergic agents, cardiovascular considerations, and the question of whether a patient with cognitive impairment can give genuinely informed consent to an intervention involving profound alteration of consciousness. Set and setting matter, and so does medical screening.

The consent question is not a clause. It is the hardest ethical problem in this section and it does not have a tidy resolution. Informed consent requires understanding the intervention, appreciating its risks as they apply to oneself, reasoning about alternatives, and communicating a choice. ABI can compromise any of these, sometimes subtly and sometimes variably across a single day. The intervention in question involves a period during which the person's capacity to withdraw consent is itself altered. And the population includes people whose distress is severe enough that they may agree to nearly anything offered as hope. None of this makes research impossible or unethical. It does mean that capacity assessment cannot be a signature on a form, and that the appropriate setting for these questions is a research protocol with ethical oversight rather than an individual clinician's judgment in an office.

Any exploration belongs in properly approved research contexts with full consent, psychiatric support, and medical oversight. Clinicians may reasonably follow this field; following is different from offering, and patients who ask should be given a clear-eyed account rather than either enthusiasm or dismissal.

8.9 Integration: What a Future Clinic Might Look Like

The original chapter offered a composite day at a future rehabilitation center: AI-guided morning priming with a neuroadaptive headset adjusting to EEG and heart rate; brain-computer-interface-assisted gait training with real-time feedback and fatigue detection; VR cognitive rehabilitation that notices frustration and inserts a regulation break before returning to task; and an AI-supported interdisciplinary team review that surfaces patterns across the week.

This vision is retained as a **thought experiment**, clearly labeled, rather than as description of current or imminent practice.

What the vignette gets right deserves attention, because it is not the technology. Every element in that day describes *attentiveness*: noticing when the patient is ready to learn, noticing fatigue before crash, noticing frustration before disengagement, and noticing patterns across a week that no single session reveals. Those are things skilled clinicians already do, imperfectly and intermittently, limited by having one set of eyes and a full caseload.

That reframing is clinically useful. It suggests that the value of these tools lies in extending clinical attention rather than substituting for it, and that a program with excellent attentiveness and modest technology will outperform a program with the reverse. It also suggests where to invest first: in the practices that make attentiveness possible, adequate session length, consistent staff, and time to think, rather than in equipment.

It also offers a test that can be applied to any new tool before purchase. Ask what clinical attention the tool extends, and whether that attention is currently missing because it is truly beyond human capacity or because the schedule does not permit it. The first is a case for technology. The second is a case for changing the schedule, and buying a device to compensate for a structural problem tends to produce an expensive version of the same problem.

A second observation about that imagined day is easy to miss. Nothing in it describes a conversation. The patient in the vignette is monitored, adjusted, and optimized, and never asked what they want their life to look like. A clinic could implement every element of that day and still deliver worse care than a well-run program with none of it, because the elements that produce durable change in ABI recovery, understanding what matters to this person, building a plan they can believe in, and staying with them while it is hard, are not among the things being automated. That is not an argument against the technology. It is an argument for noticing what a technological vision leaves out, since what a vision leaves out is usually what gets defunded first.

8.10 Guidance for Clinicians

14. **Distinguish categories rigorously.** Available now, in trials, preclinical, and speculative are different things, and most harm in this space comes from presenting one as another, usually inadvertently by someone enthusiastic.
15. **Ask what specific claim is being made.** "PEMF is supported by research" is not a claim. "This device, at these parameters, improves this outcome in this population" is, and it is usually where support thins.
16. **Stay informed without defaulting to early adoption.** New does not mean better. Patients with ABI are frequently financially strained and are targeted by marketing precisely because their condition is chronic, poorly served, and frightening.
17. **Weigh cost as a clinical variable.** Recommending an expensive device to a patient who has lost income is a clinical decision with consequences, not a neutral suggestion. Ask what else that money is for.
18. **Keep informed consent genuine.** Where something is investigational, say so plainly. Patients trust clinicians who name uncertainty more than those who do not, and that trust is the foundation of everything else.
19. **Remember the base.** Sleep, pacing, graded activity, vestibular rehabilitation, and relational care will outperform most of this chapter for most patients, and they are available today at no cost.
20. **Know what you would need to see.** For any technology you are tracking, decide in advance what evidence would change your practice: which population, which outcome, which study design. Clinicians who have not answered this question in advance tend to be moved by whichever paper they encounter most recently, or by the most confident person in the room.
21. **Track the field without letting it set the agenda.** Emerging technology is interesting, and interest is not the same as priority. The patient in front of you is more likely to be limited by unaddressed sleep disruption, unmanaged autonomic dysregulation, or an unsustainable activity pattern than by lack of access to anything in this chapter.

8.11 Where These Developments Live in the Model

Emerging technologies are easier to evaluate when they are placed inside the frameworks this book has already built, rather than treated as a separate category of thing. Placement does three useful jobs: it clarifies what a tool is actually for, it exposes what a tool cannot do regardless of how well it works, and it reveals when a clinic's enthusiasm has clustered in one part of the model while other parts go unattended.

By Realm. Recall from Chapter 1 that the Five Realms run from the most subtle to the most dense: Essence, Awareness, Field, Flow, and Form. Nearly every technology in this chapter operates in Flow or Form. Neuromodulation, PEMF, adaptive systems, and ultrasound act on physiology and regulation. VR reaches somewhat further into Awareness by working with attention and perception, and touches Field through environmental grading. Consciousness-based approaches are the exception rather than the rule, operating substantially in Awareness and, where meaning and identity are engaged, in Essence.

The pattern in that distribution is itself the finding. Technology concentrates where measurement is easiest, which is the dense end of the spectrum. Essence, the realm of identity, meaning, and coherence, is where much of the long-term suffering after brain injury actually lives, as Chapter 10 develops, and it is the realm least served by anything in this chapter. A clinic that invests heavily in emerging technology and thinly in identity, meaning, and relationship has not built a more advanced program. It has built a program that is well equipped in the part of the model that was already best served.

By Core Domain. The Five Core Domains from Chapter 3 (Energy, Metabolism, Cognition, Relationship, Environment) sort these tools by where care is directed:

Domain	Technologies from this chapter	What this reveals
Energy	PEMF and photobiomodulation development, TUS, adaptive neurofeedback	The most crowded domain; also the one where product claims most outrun product evidence
Metabolism	Little to nothing in this chapter	Emerging technology is not addressing the metabolic contributors described in Chapters 3 and 6; existing approaches remain the relevant ones
Cognition	VR and AR rehabilitation, AI-adaptive cognitive training, BCI-assisted training	Reasonable evidence for trained-task gains; transfer remains the persistent open question
Relationship	Essentially nothing	The domain most predictive of engagement and adherence is the one no device addresses

Domain	Technologies from this chapter	What this reveals
Environment	VR-graded exposure, AR overlays, remote delivery expanding access	Underused; the access gains here may matter more than the sensory ones

Two entries in that table are findings rather than as gaps to be filled. Metabolism and Relationship are not empty because those domains are unimportant. They are empty because neither is easily productized, and a field's technological attention follows what can be sold at least as closely as it follows what patients need. A clinician who notices this can compensate deliberately. A clinician who does not may drift toward whichever domain the market has equipped, and mistake that drift for progress.

By phase. The Three-Phase Model from Chapter 9 sequences care as Priming, then Intensive Neural Activation, then Reinforcement, and most of this chapter's tools belong to phase two. Adaptive systems, VR training, and neuromodulation are activation technologies: they intensify or refine demanding work. This has a direct practical consequence. Applying an activation technology to a patient who is still in Priming, before sleep, pacing, and autonomic regulation are established, tends to produce exactly the pattern described in §8.3, which is a tool recorded as ineffective when the actual problem was sequence.

Phase one is served less by new technology than by the unglamorous foundations, though remote monitoring and home-based HRV work have a legitimate role in establishing regulation. Phase three, reinforcement and generalization, is the phase where technology is weakest, because the task is transferring gains into a person's actual life, and a person's actual life is not a controllable environment. That weakness is not incidental. It reflects the same boundary the rest of this chapter keeps arriving at.

8.12 What Technology Cannot Carry

Every section of this chapter has run into the same limit from a different direction, and it should be stated directly rather than left as an implication.

Technology in rehabilitation extends measurement, repetition, precision, and access. Those are real contributions and none of them should be minimized, particularly access, which determines whether care reaches people at all. What technology does not do is decide what recovery is for. It does not sit with a person who has just understood that they will not return to the work that defined them. It does not notice that today's session should be abandoned in favor of a conversation. It does not carry the relationship through the months when progress is invisible and the patient's belief in recovery is the only thing keeping the plan alive.

These are not sentimental additions to clinical work. They are the mechanism by which the rest of the work becomes possible. Chapter 3 establishes relationship-centered care as an operating principle rather than a domain of intervention, precisely because it is the condition under which intervention functions. A patient who does not feel safe, understood, and involved in decisions will not sustain the demanding practice that produces change, regardless of how well instrumented that practice is. Adherence is not a personality trait. It is largely a product of whether the plan makes sense to the person and whether they trust the person who made it.

This gives the clinician a workable principle for the years ahead. Technology should be adopted where it removes an obstacle to attentive, individualized, relationship-centered care, and declined where it substitutes for that care or consumes the resources that make it possible. A device that frees clinician attention for the conversation is worth having. A device that fills the session so completely that the conversation never happens has cost more than it charged.

The individualization point deserves the same treatment, because it is where technology's promise and its limitation meet most directly. Adaptive systems individualize parameters within a task. That is useful and it is not what this book means by individualized care. Individualization in the sense that matters begins with what this person's life requires, what they are willing to spend their limited energy on, and what recovery would need to look like for it to count as recovery to them. No algorithm generates that. It comes from asking, and from listening carefully enough to hear an answer that may not match what the clinician expected.

Curiosity about what is coming is appropriate and this chapter has tried to model it. The field is moving, some of that movement will help patients, and clinicians who follow it will serve their patients better than those who do not. The boundary is simply that curiosity is directed at possibilities while care is delivered to a person, and the person is entitled to the truth about which is which.

Chapter 8 Quick-Reference Guide and Summary

By status.

- **Available now with reasonable evidence:** VR and AR rehabilitation (screen for vestibular and visual provocation); expectancy effects engaged through open-label rather than deceptive means; meditation and regulation practice.
- **In trials:** AI-adaptive systems and neurofeedback; transcranial ultrasound stimulation; psychedelic-assisted therapy for psychiatric indications, not ABI.

- **Emerging:** advanced PEMF protocols and photobiomodulation.
- **Speculative or unsupported:** "quantum resonance" devices (subject to regulatory action); GDV and biofield imaging as diagnostics; non-local healing claims; biophoton-based intention effects.

The four evaluative questions.

22. What is it actually doing, mechanically?
23. What clinical question would it answer?
24. What evidence exists, and in which population?
25. What would responsible adoption require?

What a measurement must demonstrate before clinical use. Reliability, validity, specificity, and responsiveness that informs a decision (§8.6).

Cross-cutting principles.

- Ask what specific claim is made, supported by what evidence, in whom.
- Distinguish modality evidence from product evidence.
- Treat cost, access, and data privacy as clinical variables.
- Extend clinical attention rather than replacing it.
- Sequence matters: an activation tool applied during Priming will often be recorded as a failed tool.
- Name uncertainty; it builds more trust than confidence does.

Where the model shows the gaps. Emerging technology clusters in Energy and Cognition, in the Flow and Form Realms, and in phase two of the Three-Phase Model. Metabolism, Relationship, and Essence remain thinly served, and phase three least served of all. Those gaps are where deliberate clinical attention matters most, because nothing in the market will fill them by default.

Chapter 9: Clinical Integration and Evolving Practice

For decades, ABI rehabilitation has been shaped by an assumption: that recovery is primarily about compensating for lost function rather than restoring it. Patients have been taught to work around deficits. This has helped many people regain mobility, communication, and independence, but it often stops short.

Many survivors find themselves at a frustrating plateau, still managing brain fog, sensory overload, autonomic instability, and cognitive fatigue long after formal rehabilitation ends. They are told progress has peaked. The evidence on plasticity suggests a more hopeful picture: the brain remains capable of change well beyond the windows once assumed, given the right conditions.

> **An honest qualification.** "The brain remains plastic for decades" is true as a statement about capacity and false if heard as a promise of continued functional gain for every patient. Some patients continue to improve years out; others reach a genuine plateau, and living well within real limitations is a legitimate and often healthier goal than indefinite pursuit of further recovery. Both messages belong in this chapter, and offering only the first one does patients harm.

9.1 Integrating QIM into Real-World Workflows

The transition does not require overhaul. It requires starting.

Begin with low-cost, high-impact interventions. HRV biofeedback and guided breathwork to support autonomic regulation. Sleep and pacing work. Targeted nutritional support. These carry the strongest evidence-to-cost ratio in the entire model and require minimal equipment.

Use monitoring where it earns its place. Wearable HRV tracking can support pacing decisions and give patients meaningful feedback. Home-based tools extend care between visits. Keep monitoring simple and sustainable; data overload is a real failure mode, and tracking that increases anxiety should be scaled back.

Shift toward interdisciplinary practice. Hold regular case reviews incorporating functional findings, relevant biomarkers, and therapy progress. Cross-train across disciplines so that a speech-language pathologist understands autonomic regulation and a physician understands what rehabilitation therapists are actually doing.

> **Action Step: Ways to provide integrative care.** Start with one intervention, one patient population, and one measurable outcome. Document what happens. Expand what works; drop what does not. This is more persuasive to colleagues and administrators than enthusiasm, and it protects patients from your own untested assumptions.

9.2 Improving Outcomes Through Collaboration

Recovery will not remain siloed. The most effective programs combine neurology, rehabilitation therapies, mental health, nutrition, and regulation-focused practice, with genuine communication rather than parallel documentation.

Practical collaboration means shared language about goals, agreement on who is tracking what, and explicit handoffs. It also means tolerating disagreement: a physician skeptical of a modality and a therapist enthusiastic about it can still coordinate well if both are honest about evidence and both keep the patient's priorities central.

9.3 Aligning Technology, Teams, and Tools

Technology should serve the plan, not generate it. Before adding any tool, ask what clinical question it answers, whether that question changes management, whether the patient can sustain its use, and what it costs them in money, time, and attention.

The same applies to the model as a whole. The Five Core Domains (Chapter 3) tell you where to work. The Three-Phase Model (below) tells you when. Tools fill in the how, and they are the most replaceable element.

9.4 The Three-Phase Model: Sequencing Care

Priming, then Intensive Neural Activation, then Reinforcement is presented as **Dr. Sarah Young's clinical-organizing framework, an original translational synthesis for sequencing ABI care**. Individual components carry their own evidence labels, developed in Chapter 4; the sequencing itself is clinical reasoning rather than an independently validated protocol, and it is offered as such.

Phase one: Priming. Establishing readiness before more demanding work begins. Aerobic exercise is included in guideline recommendations for persistent post-concussion symptoms, although the recommendations are weak and based on low to very low certainty evidence (Rytter et al., 2021). Sleep, pacing, autonomic regulation, and metabolic support belong here. The phase's purpose is to make the next phase possible rather than to produce gains directly.

Phase two: Intensive Neural Activation. The demanding work: task-specific training, dual-task integration, action-observation and motor imagery, cognitive rehabilitation. This is where the strongest conventional rehabilitation evidence lives (Cicerone et al., 2019; Kleim & Jones, 2008), and integrative work should support it rather than compete with it.

Phase three: Reinforcement. Consolidation and generalization: transferring gains into real-world contexts, metacognitive strategy training (Kennedy et al., 2008), and sustainable routines. Skills that do not generalize have not really been gained.

The phases are not rigid stages. Patients move between them, and different domains may sit in different phases simultaneously: a patient may be in Reinforcement for mobility and still in Priming for cognitive load tolerance.

CASE EXAMPLE

Marcus, Continued: Sequencing and Integration

The same fictional educational composite, shown here as a full arc, not a real patient or real treatment record.

Looking back across the whole span of Marcus's care, from the first attempts at recognizing his autonomic pattern through the later work on his gut symptoms, shows something the individual episodes don't: how much the sequence itself shaped what happened, not just which tools eventually got used. Each phase built directly on what the previous one had already established rather than introducing everything at once. Early on, there was no way to know whether starting differently would have gotten him somewhere similar, faster, or whether the graduated approach itself was doing real work.

Read in order, his care looks like a deliberate structure rather than a pile of unrelated interventions: foundational, low-burden work first, then more active regulation tools, then the later additions. At every layer, the priority was the same, confirm tolerance and settle on a clear clinical question before adding anything new, so tools entered his care deliberately rather than all together. Accessible, easily-monitored strategies came first, so his early response could actually be seen. Technology-assisted tools came in once a specific question justified them. Gut-directed changes arrived one at a time, only once his autonomic picture had stabilized enough that a new variable could mean something. None of this reflected an assumption that anything added later mattered less than what came first; it reflected what could actually be tracked at each stage.

His trajectory across the whole period was gradual and layered, not a single turning point anyone could point to. And there's a real limit here: no single composite case can say how much the sequencing itself mattered, versus the simple cumulative effect of the tools involved.

What this illustrates is why order and pacing deserve real attention in a multi-system recovery, not just the choice of intervention. What it cannot do is prove that the three-phase sequencing model outperforms another approach. It shows the reasoning behind sequencing, not a controlled comparison.

9.5 Patient-Facing Tracking Tools

Simple, sustainable tracking supports both clinical decisions and patient insight. General symptom, mood, and habit tracking applications work well for many patients, as do purpose-built recovery and mindfulness applications, several of which are available at no cost through veterans' health services and are worth knowing about for cost-constrained patients. Appendix A provides structured tracking tools that do not require any technology.

Match the tool to the person. A patient with executive-function difficulty needs fewer fields, not more. A patient prone to health anxiety may need tracking reduced or paused. Detailed guidance on data literacy and its risks appears in Chapter 6.

Chapter 9 Quick-Reference Guide and Summary

- **Start small:** low-cost, high-evidence interventions first, with one measurable outcome.
- **Plateau honesty:** continued plasticity is real; guaranteed continued gain is not, and adaptation is a legitimate goal.
- **Collaboration:** shared language, explicit ownership, tolerance for principled disagreement.
- **Three-Phase Model:** Priming, Intensive Neural Activation, Reinforcement, as the author's sequencing synthesis, complementing the Five Core Domains.
- **Tools serve plans:** ask what question a tool answers and what it costs the patient before adopting it.

Chapter 10: Quantum Medicine in Action

Healing from brain injury does not only require the right tools. It requires the right clinician. The therapeutic relationship, the way we communicate, and the flexibility of our approach are not extras layered on top of technique; they determine whether technique lands at all.

This chapter is about the practitioner. It addresses attunement, adaptive communication, self-awareness, and honest innovation, and it does so on the premise that in ABI care these are clinical skills with measurable consequences rather than matters of personal style. It is not only what you do. It is how you show up, and for patients whose nervous systems are reading the room continuously, how you show up is part of the intervention.

10.1 Health Literacy as an Act of Healing

Health literacy goes far beyond understanding medical terminology. For patients recovering from ABI it means navigating information while managing memory difficulty, slowed processing, and trouble sequencing, often while frightened and often while being handed more information than anyone could absorb.

In this context clinicians are educators, and translators as well. Our task is converting complex information into something usable, and the measure of success is not whether we explained it well but whether the patient can act on it tomorrow.

The teach-back method is the most effective tool available. Rather than assuming understanding, invite patients to restate: "Can you tell me what you took from that?" This surfaces confusion while you can still address it. The framing matters enormously: asked as a check on your own clarity, "I want to make sure I explained that well," it protects dignity. Asked as a quiz, it humiliates.

Pairing visual and verbal information engages more channels and supports retention. Simple flowcharts, dry-erase sketches, icons, and written summaries frequently outperform paragraphs of careful prose. Many clinicians find that drawing while explaining slows their own pace usefully and gives the patient something to take home.

Practical adaptations that matter. Limit new information per visit; two remembered points beat six forgotten. Put the most important thing first and repeat it last. Provide written summaries in plain language rather than clinical shorthand. Invite the patient to record the explanation on their phone, which many find transformative and few think to ask for. Include caregivers with permission, and check what the caregiver understood too.

A note on tone. Patients with cognitive impairment are often spoken to either too simply, which is demeaning, or at normal complexity, which excludes them. The target is ordinary adult language delivered slowly, with structure, and with real checking. Simplify the syntax, not the respect.

10.2 Emotional Intelligence and Therapeutic Presence

Emotional intelligence lets us perceive what a patient is experiencing beneath what they are saying and respond to that rather than to the surface. It helps us recognize that what looks like resistance may be fear, that silence may signal cognitive overload rather than disagreement, and that irritability may be grief, exhaustion, or the accumulated frustration of not being believed.

Practicing this begins with awareness of the patient's state and, equally, of our own. Pausing before correcting creates room to respond rather than react. A validating statement, "It makes sense you would feel that way," can open a door that persuasion cannot. **Validation is not agreement; it is acknowledgment**, and the distinction gives clinicians permission to validate an experience while disagreeing with an interpretation, which Chapter 7's EMF discussion requires.

Asking about emotional patterns builds metacognitive skill. "Have you noticed this comes up more when you are tired?" respects the patient's self-knowledge and helps them connect internal states with behavior, which is the foundation of self-regulation and something many patients have lost access to after injury.

Regulating ourselves is the most overlooked strategy and possibly the most consequential. Patients with ABI are frequently hypersensitive to tone, pace, and nonverbal cues, in part because injury heightens threat detection and in part because they have learned to read clinicians for signs of dismissal. A clinician who is rushed communicates that regardless of what they say. Showing up settled offers a co-regulatory presence that the patient's nervous system can organize around, which is a real physiological effect rather than a metaphor.

This has a practical implication: your own regulation is part of your clinical preparation. Two minutes between patients is not indulgence; it is the difference between offering regulation and transmitting urgency.

Trauma-informed care builds on this foundation. Many survivors carry layered trauma: from the injury itself, from emergency and hospital care, from the loss of role and capacity, and frequently from before the injury. Trauma-informed practice means predictable routines, genuine choices, avoiding power struggles, explaining before doing, and centering agency. SAMHSA's framework, safety, trustworthiness and transparency, peer support, collaboration, empowerment, and attention to cultural and historical context (SAMHSA, 2014), provides the standard reference and translates directly to this setting.

One specific application deserves emphasis: **do not require patients to prove their symptoms before receiving help.** Many arrive expecting to have to, and releasing them from that expectation changes what they are able to tell you.

10.3 Adaptive, Personalized Practice

Patients differ in how they take in information, and after ABI those differences sharpen into access requirements. Some need visual structure. Some do better narrating routines aloud. Some need to move through a task physically before they can describe it. These are neurological access points rather than preferences, and getting them wrong wastes sessions.

Emotional and sensory thresholds deserve equal respect. Sensory overload, fatigue, and emotional lability can derail a session that was well planned. Embedding regulation cues, pacing deliberately, and checking in periodically make therapy feel manageable rather than punishing. Some patients benefit from a weighted item, noise-reducing headphones, dimmed lighting, or a visually quiet space. Others need short bursts of activity with real rest between rather than a continuous forty-five minutes.

Reading the moment matters as much as the plan. A patient arriving dysregulated may need grounding before anything else, and the ten minutes spent there frequently buys the remaining thirty. A patient arriving with unusual energy may be ready for the demanding task you had deferred, and taking that opening is better practice than following the schedule.

This is not permission to improvise indefinitely. The plan provides direction and accountability; the moment determines the route.

> **Clinician Tip: Treat the plan as a guide, not a script.** Observe learning style, emotional state, and energy in real time. Ask yourself: how is this person taking in information today? Do they need regulation before we begin, or are they ready to engage? Then ask them, because they often know.

10.4 Case Snapshots: What the Composite Arcs Show

The composite cases introduced in Chapter 5 are drawn on throughout this book. Read as complete arcs rather than as episodes, they illustrate what this chapter is describing.

Marcus shows the value of sequencing. His care began with autonomic pattern recognition, moved through gastrointestinal symptoms considered within a broader picture rather than as an isolated complaint, and later addressed integration across his whole course. What his arc demonstrates is not that any single intervention worked but that order mattered: foundational, low-burden work first, then more active regulation, then additions once he had capacity for them. It also demonstrates the honest limit, since no composite can establish how much the sequencing itself contributed versus the components or simply time.

Priya shows how a premature explanation can obscure a fuller picture without being wrong. Her fog and fatigue were attributed to depression and to ordinary recovery. Her sadness was real; it was also incomplete as an account. The clinical work was holding both, pursuing physiological contributors without dismissing the psychological ones, and treating them concurrently rather than in sequence.

Theo shows the arc from safety to identity. Early work established enough regulation and trust for him to engage at all. Later work addressed something no functional measure captures: who he understood himself to be after injury, and whether that person had a future he wanted.

These are disclosed fictional educational composites, not case reports. They illustrate reasoning. They cannot establish efficacy, causation, or response rates, and this book's effectiveness claims rest on the cited literature and its evidence labels rather than on these narratives.

CASE EXAMPLE

Theo, Continued: Identity Over the Long Arc

Theo's composite story continues, several years further along, the same fictional educational composite, not a real patient or real treatment history.

Several years out from his injury, about two years past the shift in his care described earlier, Theo's functional symptoms had settled into a long-term pattern he'd learned to work with. They hadn't disappeared. Most of his earlier care, understandably, had chased symptom management and functional goals: walk further, remember more, manage the fatigue. But somewhere along the way a different question surfaced, one nobody had quite named yet. What did "recovery" actually mean for him now? A full return to who he'd been before wasn't realistic, and building his whole sense of self around what he'd lost didn't fit his experience either. Neither story was true.

So the conversations turned toward identity directly: what mattered to him now, what continuity he still felt with the person he'd been, what had genuinely changed, without assuming the answer had to be loss on one side or triumphant reinvention on the other. The work that followed was relational and reflective rather than protocol-driven, ongoing conversation, room to grieve what had changed, space to notice what he valued now that had never been part of his life before. The aim throughout was holding continuity, loss, adaptation, and emerging possibility together, rather than pushing him toward "getting back to normal" or toward an entirely reinvented story of who he was.

Something did shift. Theo started describing himself less as someone failing to return to a former version of himself, and more as someone shaped by his injury without being defined by it. It's a change in his relationship to his own experience, not a resolution of it. His physical and cognitive symptoms are still part of his daily life. There's no clean endpoint where this work gets to call itself finished.

This composite shows that long-term adaptation after brain injury can be a real, meaningful outcome even without symptom resolution, and that identity work isn't a return to who someone was or the construction of someone entirely new. It doesn't represent a typical timeline, and it shouldn't be read as suggesting identity integration follows a predictable course toward a fixed endpoint. For most people, it won't.

10.5 Practitioner and Patient Perspectives

Two perspectives sit at the center of this work, and holding both is most of the skill.

From the practitioner's side, integrative work requires tolerance of uncertainty that conventional training does not always cultivate. You will use interventions whose evidence is incomplete. You will be asked questions you cannot answer definitively, by people who need an answer. The sustainable posture is to say what is established, what is promising, and what you do not know, and to be equally clear about all three.

This is more protective than it sounds. Clinicians who overclaim eventually meet the patient for whom it did not work, and that patient loses faith in the intervention, in the clinician, and often in the whole approach. Clinicians who state uncertainty accurately find that a failed intervention costs them nothing, because they never promised otherwise.

There is also a harder truth about this work: it exposes you to a great deal of suffering that you cannot fix. Patients with ABI frequently do not fully recover. Sitting with that, without either detaching or absorbing it, is a skill that requires deliberate maintenance. Supervision, peer consultation, and your own regulation practice are not optional extras for a clinician doing this work over years.

From the patient's side, the most consistent theme across ABI narratives is not any intervention. It is the experience of not being believed. Invisible symptoms, unremarkable imaging, and fluctuating capacity combine so that patients feel they must prove their difficulty before receiving help. Many have been told their fatigue is depression, their dizziness is anxiety, their fog is stress. Some of these were partly true; delivered without curiosity, all of them taught the patient that describing symptoms produces dismissal.

The consequences are practical. Patients arrive defensive, or overstate certainty because tentativeness has invited dismissal, or omit symptoms they expect to be doubted. A clinician who begins from belief has already changed what information they will receive.

The convergence. Take symptoms entirely seriously. Hold explanations lightly. Be honest about uncertainty in both directions, about what you do not know and about what the evidence does not support. And stay in the relationship long enough for the work to answer questions that argument cannot.

10.6 Barriers and Adaptations

Real barriers shape what any of this can accomplish, and naming them is more useful than a model that assumes ideal conditions.

Cost and coverage. Many integrative interventions are not reimbursed. Patients frequently lose income precisely when expenses rise. An enthusiastic clinician can do genuine harm by recommending devices, supplements, and testing a family cannot afford but will attempt anyway, sometimes at the expense of necessities. **A version of this care that costs nothing should always be available and should be offered first:** sleep, light timing, pacing, breathwork, hydration, movement, environmental modification, and education carry much of the available benefit.

Geographic access. Trained practitioners cluster in metropolitan areas. Telehealth addresses part of this, and much of the highest-value work translates well to remote delivery. Where specialists are unavailable, clinicians can often supervise foundational work themselves rather than referring indefinitely into a void.

Cognitive load as a barrier to care itself. This is the cruelest structural feature of ABI: navigating fragmented healthcare requires exactly the executive function the injury impaired. Patients miss appointments, cannot track referrals, and abandon processes that a well person would complete. Adaptations matter: written summaries, appointment reminders, help with scheduling, coordinating rather than multiplying referrals, and involving a support person with permission. Reducing the administrative burden of receiving care is itself clinical work.

Fluctuating capacity. A patient who managed last month may not manage this month. Build plans with a floor version, the minimum that preserves progress on a bad week, so that a hard stretch does not become a full stop.

Family and social context. Recovery happens inside relationships that the injury has also strained. Caregivers burn out, roles shift, and financial pressure alters what is possible. Asking about this directly changes what plans are realistic.

10.7 Future-Facing Practice

The clinician's role is shifting as the tools change. Chapter 8 surveys what is coming; this section addresses what it asks of us.

Increasingly, we will be asked to interpret data rather than only to observe: HRV trends, tracking logs, adaptive system outputs. That requires comfort with pattern recognition and with the limits of measurement, including the discipline to say that a number does not mean what a patient hopes it means.

We will be asked about interventions before evidence exists, because patients find them first. The useful stance is neither gatekeeping nor enthusiasm but honest triage: what is this, what is claimed, what is supported, what would it cost you, and what would we watch for.

We will work in teams that cross traditional boundaries, which requires the ability to explain our reasoning to people who do not share our framework and to hear theirs.

And through all of it, the elements that matter most are the ones least likely to be automated: presence, judgment, the ability to sit with uncertainty, and the willingness to be affected by another person's situation without being destabilized by it.

10.8 The Clinician as the Instrument

Being an integrative clinician means showing up with both skill and heart: speaking to empower rather than overwhelm, reframing limitations as evolving capacities without minimizing real loss, and using both data and judgment. It means co-regulating before educating, listening before instructing, and tailoring each moment to the nervous system in front of you.

When we communicate adaptively, our work becomes accessible. When we mark real progress, however small, we reinforce it. When we support patients to observe, track, and direct their own recovery, we help them reclaim agency in a process that has often felt entirely beyond their control.

The most important element in the room is not the device, the protocol, or the program.

Chapter 10 Quick-Reference Guide and Summary

Core concepts.

- **Health literacy as intervention:** teach-back framed as a check on your clarity, visual-verbal pairing, limited information per visit, ordinary adult language delivered slowly.
- **Emotional intelligence:** validation without agreement, pattern inquiry, clinician self-regulation as clinical preparation, trauma-informed practice per SAMHSA's six principles, and never requiring patients to prove their symptoms.
- **Adaptive practice:** read the moment alongside the plan, respect sensory and emotional thresholds, treat learning style as an access requirement.
- **Case snapshots:** Marcus (sequencing), Priya (incomplete explanations), Theo (safety to identity), all disclosed composites illustrating reasoning rather than evidence.
- **Two perspectives:** clinician tolerance of uncertainty and sustainable exposure to suffering; patient experience of not being believed.
- **Barriers:** cost, geography, cognitive load as a barrier to care itself, fluctuating capacity, family context, with a no-cost version always offered first.
- **Future-facing practice:** interpreting data honestly, triaging novelty, working across frameworks, and retaining what cannot be automated.

Chapter 11: Closing Reflections: The Future Is Integrative

The future of rehabilitation is not built on rigid protocols but on integration: of systems, of science and soul, of brain and body, of practitioner and patient. At the heart of Quantum Integrative Medicine for Acquired Brain Injury is a simple truth: healing is not linear, and recovery cannot be reduced to symptoms and checklists. True healing asks for coherence across every layer of a person's being: physical, energetic, emotional, cognitive, and in their sense of self.

Throughout this guide, you have explored what it means to treat the whole person. You have been invited to see beyond diagnosis, to listen through a trauma-informed lens, to use clinical tools that regulate the nervous system, support neuroplasticity, restore gut-brain balance, and open space for emotional and consciousness-based healing. But this work cannot be reduced to charts and figures. Its power lies in how you embody it. You are not simply applying a model; in a real sense you are the model in motion, practicing presence, curiosity, humility, and deep care. Whenever you choose connection over correction, curiosity over judgment, and relationship over routine, you redefine what is possible in clinical care.

Quantum Integrative Medicine is not a fixed destination. It is an unfolding path that invites you to keep learning, refining, and adapting with every person you serve. It asks us to let go of "fixing" and to step into facilitation, collaboration, and empowerment. As you move forward, know this: you are not alone. You are part of a growing community of clinicians, coaches, and consciousness-informed healers who believe in the body's ability to recover, the brain's capacity to rewire, and the heart's power to guide the process.

The future of medicine is not one-size-fits-all. The future is relational. The future is neuroplastic. The future is integrative. And it starts with how you show up today.

Thank you for doing this work. The world needs your wisdom, warmth, and willingness to reimagine what is possible.

Appendices

The five appendices that follow are practical companions to the chapters. Appendix A supports tracking, Appendix B supports staff training, Appendix C maps symptoms to intervention categories, Appendix D supports referral and resource decisions, and Appendix E offers sample protocols.

Appendix A: Tools for Tracking Neuroplastic and Physiological Improvement

This appendix offers a toolkit for assessing, monitoring, and tracking progress in QIM-based ABI rehabilitation, organized by domain. Two principles govern its use: **introduce one tool at a time**, matched to the patient's tolerance and cognitive load; and **track what will change a decision**, since tracking that does not inform care adds burden without benefit.

A.1 Neuroplasticity and Cognitive Function

Standardized cognitive assessment. The NIH Toolbox Cognition Battery measures memory, attention, executive function, and processing speed. Use at baseline with periodic follow-up. It is standardized, efficient, and reasonably sensitive to change. *(Well validated.)*

Goal Attainment Scaling (GAS). Measures individualized, patient-defined goals across motor, cognitive, and emotional domains at baseline and at intervals. GAS deserves more prominence than it usually receives: it captures what matters to the patient rather than only what is easy to measure, and it has genuine support in rehabilitation settings. *(Well validated.)*

Digital cognitive training platforms. BrainHQ and **Lumosity** track reaction time, memory, attention, and visual processing, with exportable progress data suitable for review in session. BrainHQ has more published supporting work than most competitors. *(Evidence label: improvement on a training platform reliably demonstrates improvement at that platform's tasks; transfer to real-world function is much weaker and should not be implied to patients. Marketing in this sector has been subject to regulatory action historically. Use as engagement and practice tools, not outcome measures. Consumer wellness; subscription-based, pricing changes frequently.)*

A.2 Autonomic and Regulatory Function

Heart rate variability monitoring. Daily or session-based tracking of vagal tone, stress recovery, and regulation trends. HRV is among the most practical repeatable measures in this model. Commonly used tools include the **Oura Ring** and **WHOOP** (passive overnight capture, minimal user effort, well suited to executive-function difficulty), **Elite HRV** with a chest strap (more accurate beat-to-beat measurement than optical sensors), **HeartMath Inner Balance** (real-time coherence training rather than passive tracking), and **Apple Watch** or **Fitbit** (broader tracking, lower entry cost). *(Evidence label: modality evidence for HRV as an autonomic marker is reasonable and ABI-relevant. Product evidence is thin:*

no consumer device has ABI-specific outcome data, accuracy varies substantially by sensor type, and chest-strap ECG outperforms wrist and finger optical sensors for beat-to-beat variability. Trends within one device are meaningful; absolute values and cross-device comparison are not. Consumer wellness, clinician-interpreted. Most carry subscriptions; verify current cost, which is a recurring burden for patients who have lost income.)

Quantitative EEG. Measures brainwave patterns and coherence, used at longer intervals. Apply the constraints stated throughout this book: qEEG findings are not specific to TBI, are influenced by alertness, sleep, medication, and analytic method, and should not independently establish diagnosis, determine severity, or prescribe a neurofeedback protocol. *(Limited as an outcome measure.)*

A.3 Metabolic and Neuroimmune Function

Inflammatory markers such as hs-CRP and IL-6 may be tracked periodically to follow systemic inflammatory status. *(Population-level indicators; no single marker identifies the cause of an individual patient's symptoms.)*

Organic acids and metabolic panels are used in functional practice to explore mitochondrial and oxidative status. *(Evidence label: these panels have significant validation limitations for the interpretive claims commonly made from them, and they are expensive. Order them when a specific clinical question requires them, not routinely, and interpret conservatively. Appendix D's pre-test checklist applies.)*

A.4 Emotional and Psychological Recovery

PHQ-9 and GAD-7 track depression and anxiety severity at regular intervals. These are well validated, free, brief, and clinically essential in this population, where mood symptoms are common, treatable, and frequently attributed entirely to the injury. **Any concerning score, particularly on PHQ-9 item nine, requires direct clinical follow-up rather than tracking alone.**

Perceived Stress Scale tracks subjective stress burden, useful for correlating experience with physiological measures.

NeuroSynergy Self-Perception Journal. A structured daily or weekly reflection tracking energy, clarity, mood, and observations. Its value is less as measurement than as a support for self-awareness and for richer clinician-patient conversation.

A.4a Recommended Applications and Digital Resources

Named here because several are **free and publicly funded**, which makes them among the most practical recommendations available for cost-constrained patients.

Purpose-built recovery applications (US Department of Veterans Affairs, free). CBT-i Coach provides structured support for cognitive behavioral therapy for insomnia, the first-line treatment for chronic insomnia and one with real access barriers, which makes a free structured tool especially valuable. **Concussion Coach** offers symptom management tools specific to this population. **PTSD Coach** provides mood tracking and grounding techniques. **Mindfulness Coach** delivers guided practice. *(Category: consumer wellness, publicly developed. These support rather than replace clinician guidance.)*

Symptom and mood tracking. Bearable tracks symptoms, mood, and lifestyle factors together, which suits the multi-symptom picture typical after ABI. **Daylio** offers low-friction mood and activity logging requiring minimal typing, useful when writing is effortful. **Reflectly** provides guided journaling with prompts. **Tally** tracks simple habits such as hydration or practice adherence. *(Evidence label: these are conveniences that support adherence and pattern visibility, not validated instruments. Consumer wellness; free tiers vary in usefulness.)*

Meditation and regulation. Insight Timer offers a large free library of guided practice, breathwork, and sound-based sessions. **10% Happier** provides structured mindfulness training on subscription. **NeuroCycle** follows a structured reflective protocol. *(Consumer wellness. Evidence supports mindfulness and breath-based regulation as modalities; no specific application has ABI outcome data.)*

Tinnitus and auditory support. Sound-therapy applications, including those distributed by hearing-device manufacturers such as **ReSound Tinnitus Relief**, provide structured sound therapy, which has better support for tinnitus distress than supplementation does. *(Best used alongside audiology input.)*

Biofeedback and neurofeedback devices. HeartMath Inner Balance for HRV coherence training, **Muse** for consumer EEG-based meditation feedback, and **Apollo Neuro** for patterned vibration intended to influence autonomic state. *(Evidence label: HRV biofeedback as a modality has reasonable support; HeartMath's supporting literature is substantially produced by the affiliated institute, which is worth weighing. Consumer EEG headbands use few electrodes, are not equivalent to clinical EEG, and should never be presented as brain assessment. Apollo Neuro's evidence is preliminary. Consumer wellness; clinical neurofeedback by contrast is clinician-directed and requires certification.)*

A.5 Suggested Use Timeline

Tool	Domain	Typical frequency
NIH Toolbox	Cognitive function	Periodic (monthly to quarterly)
HRV monitoring	Autonomic function	Daily or per session
Inflammatory markers	Metabolic and immune	Quarterly, if clinically indicated
PHQ-9, GAD-7, PSS	Emotional health	Monthly
qEEG	Neurophysiological	Infrequent; only if it changes management
Goal Attainment Scaling	Functional goals	Baseline and monthly
Cognitive training platforms	Practice and engagement	Weekly
Self-perception journal	Self-awareness	Daily or weekly

A.6 Self-Tracking Tools

Self-tracking gives patients a tangible way to observe their own recovery, supporting autonomy and letting both patient and clinician correlate symptoms with interventions. It maps naturally onto the Five Bodies and the Five Pillars.

- **Symptom diaries.** Daily severity of headaches, dizziness, sleep, fatigue, and fog, ideally alongside notes on activity and stressors.
- **Mood logs.** Paper or app-based tracking of mood shifts, triggers, and what helped.
- **Health passports.** Personalized summaries of history, current protocols, preferences, and communication needs, valuable during care transitions and urgent visits.
- **Brain-body scoreboards.** Simple visual charts tracking consistency across daily self-care practices. Low-tech versions work well for patients with executive-function difficulty.

Integration into clinical work. Review logs at each visit to identify trends, adjust for real-world stressors, reinforce the patient's active role, and align interventions with what the patient actually reports.

> **Clinician Tip.** Introduce one tracking tool at a time. Keep it simple, visual, and tied to the patient's goals. If tracking becomes a source of anxiety or another failure to manage, reduce or stop it. See Chapter 6 on data literacy.

Appendix B: Clinician and Staff Training for Trauma-Informed, Health-Literate Care

Section 1: Building Communication and Clinical Skill

1. Communication-Partner Skills Practice

Purpose: Build concrete skill in supporting a patient who uses augmentative or alternative communication (AAC), without requiring staff to imitate the impairment itself.

Exercise: In pairs, one person plays a patient using a communication board (provided, not self-made under time pressure) to express a realistic clinical scenario, describing pain location, refusing a treatment, or asking a question. The other practices being an effective **communication partner**: asking yes/no questions when helpful, allowing full time for a response without filling silence, confirming understanding before moving on, and avoiding speaking *for* the patient. Roles switch.

Debrief: Focus on what made the "clinician" role effective or ineffective as a communication partner, specific behaviors, not personal frustration. Close with each participant naming one concrete practice they'll use in their next patient interaction (e.g., "I will wait a full 10 seconds before rephrasing a question").

2. Case-Based Communication Design

Purpose: Build skill in designing patient communication that accounts for memory and processing-speed differences, without requiring staff to simulate cognitive impairment.

Exercise: Present a real or composite case: a patient with documented short-term memory difficulty and slowed processing speed needs to be given multi-step discharge instructions. In small groups, staff redesign the instructions, chunking steps, building in confirmation checkpoints, deciding what needs to be written down versus said aloud, and planning for a follow-up call.

Debrief: Compare the redesigned instruction sets across groups. Discuss what design choices support retention and reduce cognitive load, and how to recognize when a patient may need this kind of accommodation even when it isn't stated outright.

3. Environmental Audit and Patient Narrative

Purpose: Build awareness of how a clinical space itself affects patients with sensory sensitivity, grounded in real patient experience rather than staff simulation.

Exercise: Two components, either or both depending on time: (a) **Environmental audit**, in small groups, walk through your own clinical space with a structured checklist (lighting type and brightness, background noise sources, visual clutter, wait-area predictability) and identify specific, fixable friction points. (b) **Patient narrative**, the facilitator selects a first-person account of sensory overload in a healthcare setting to share with the group, using the following criteria:

- First-person perspective from a person with ABI
- Appropriate permission for use, or a lawfully published source
- Focus on healthcare access or sensory experience specifically
- Avoids framing that invites inspiration, pity, or a deficit-only view of the person
- Ends with, or prompts discussion toward, concrete changes to clinical practice

A published first-person ABI account, a recorded narrative used with explicit permission, or a clearly labeled composite educational scenario (when no suitable first-person source is available) all satisfy these criteria, a composite should never be presented as an authentic patient testimony. If a published narrative is used, respect its permissions and any quotation limits rather than reproducing it beyond what's allowed.

Debrief: Convert audit findings into a short list of concrete environmental changes, connected to Chapter 7 §7.3's accommodation options.

4. Mirror Therapy as a Clinical Technique

Purpose: Understand mirror therapy as a specific rehabilitation technique with defined indications, not as a general demonstration of brain-based learning.

Training content: Mirror therapy has documented use for specific indications (e.g., certain motor rehabilitation and some pain conditions), with defined protocols, evidence that varies by indication, precautions, and a need for appropriately trained clinical oversight. This is training content, a short overview of what mirror therapy is, who it's appropriate for, and where to refer or seek further training, rather than a paired staff activity, since presenting it as a casual pairing exercise risked implying more mechanistic certainty ("mirror neurons" as the explanation) than the evidence actually supports.

Section 2: Health Literacy in Practice

5. Teach-Back Training Circles, Pair up and role-play patient education; the "clinician" delivers information, the "patient" paraphrases it. Debrief on clarity, pacing, and confirmation technique.

6. The 60-Second Metaphor Challenge, Staff have 60 seconds to explain a medical concept using an everyday metaphor. Debrief on which metaphors supported comprehension and why.

7. Jargon Translation Workshop, Rewrite a list of jargon terms in plain language suitable for a 6th-grade reading level. Debrief on patterns in language complexity; build a shared plain-language glossary.

8. Accessible Materials Design Lab, Review or create a patient handout with visuals, step-by-step breakdowns, and simple language. Debrief on readability and visual clarity.

Section 3: Common Medical Metaphors for ABI Patient Education

Metaphors can make complex information easier to understand and remember. They are teaching tools, not literal descriptions of biology. Ask the patient whether a metaphor fits their experience rather than assuming the same image will work for everyone.

Medical concept	Patient-friendly metaphor
Neuroplasticity	"Your brain is like a network of trails. The routes you practice become easier to travel, while new routes can develop through repetition and support."
Dysautonomia	"Your body's automatic control system is like a thermostat that has become overly sensitive. It may react strongly to standing, heat, exertion, or stress, even when the situation does not seem demanding."
Inflammation	"Think of inflammation like a fire alarm that keeps sounding after the immediate danger has passed. The goal is not to remove the alarm, but to help it respond appropriately."
Energy crisis after TBI	"Your brain is working with a smaller battery while facing higher energy demands. Pacing helps prevent it from spending tomorrow's energy today."
Gut-brain axis	"Your gut and brain are connected by a busy two-way communication line. Changes at either end can affect the messages traveling between them."
HRV and vagal tone	"Your autonomic nervous system works like a car with an accelerator and brakes. Regulation practices help it shift more smoothly instead of getting stuck pressing one pedal."
Neurofeedback	"Neurofeedback is like giving the brain a mirror. The feedback helps it notice patterns and practice shifting them over time."
ABI recovery	"Healing after brain injury can resemble rebuilding a city after a storm. First, we stabilize essential systems. Then we repair routes, reconnect services, and gradually restore capacity."

> **Clinical Application: Check the Fit.** After offering a metaphor, ask, "Does that description fit what this feels like for you?" If it does not, invite the patient to modify it or create a different comparison. The most useful metaphor is the one that increases understanding without oversimplifying or overriding the patient's experience.

Additional Recommendations

Interdisciplinary case review meetings using patient-friendly language, a shared clinic-wide "Communication Toolkit," and inviting an ABI survivor to speak directly to staff about their lived experience. That last one matters most: direct engagement with a survivor's own account teaches more than any simulation of impairment can.

Appendix C: Integrative ABI Symptom Navigation Matrix

How to use this matrix. Locate the symptom, consider the likely contributing systems, then review the intervention categories. This is a navigation aid supporting clinical reasoning, not a prescribing tool. Interventions listed are candidates to consider, weigh, and individualize, not recommendations to apply. Evidence strength varies considerably across entries; consult the relevant chapter for the labeled discussion.

Symptom	Likely contributing systems	Intervention categories to consider	System category	Chapter
Brain fog, slowed processing	Metabolic, inflammatory, sleep, autonomic	Sleep optimization, pacing, metabolic support, graded cognitive work	Energy / cognitive	2, 7
Persistent fatigue	HPA and circadian, mitochondrial, autonomic	Pacing (first-line), sleep, graded aerobic activity, adaptogens with interaction check	Energy / cellular	7
Headaches	Cervical, vascular, medication overuse, hydration, sleep	Cervical assessment, medication-overuse screening, magnesium, hydration, trigger review	Vascular / musculoskeletal	7

Symptom	Likely contributing systems	Interventio n categories to consider	System category	Chapter
Dizziness, visual strain	Vestibular, oculomotor, autonomic	**Vestibular and neuro-optometric referral (priority)**, gaze stabilization, graded exposure	Sensory / vestibular	7
Anxiety, panic	Autonomic, limbic, trauma-related	Breathwork, HRV biofeedback, trauma-informed care, mental health referral	Autonomic / limbic	4, 7, 10
Low mood, apathy	Mood disorder, dopaminergic, social isolation	**Depression screening (PHQ-9)**, behavioral activation, light exposure, movement, referral	Neuropsychiatric	7, A
Sleep disruption	Circadian, neuroendocrine, sleep-disordered breathing, pain	**Sleep apnea screening**, CBT-I, light timing, wind-down routine, melatonin for circadian issues	Circadian / neuroendocrine	7

Symptom	Likely contributing systems	Intervention categories to consider	System category	Chapter
GI symptoms, bloating	Gut-brain axis, vagal, dietary	Red-flag screening first, fiber and mucosal support, strain-appropriate probiotics, vagal work	Gastrointestinal	2, 6, 7
Hormonal or metabolic changes	Pituitary, thyroid, gonadal, adrenal axes	**Post-traumatic hypopituitarism screening per guidance; endocrinology referral**	Endocrine	7
Sound sensitivity, tinnitus	Auditory processing, limbic	Audiology referral, graded sound exposure (not avoidance), CBT-based approaches for tinnitus	Sensory / auditory	7
Chronic pain	Central sensitization, musculoskeletal, emotional	Pain neuroscience education, graded activity, somatic work, topical and botanical supports	Pain / neurologic	7
Mitochondrial and oxidative burden	Cellular energy, redox	Sleep, movement, nutrition, mitochondrial cofactors, photobiomodulation	Energy / cellular	3, 7

Symptom	Likely contributing systems	Intervention categories to consider	System category	Chapter
Sensory overload	Sensory integration, autonomic	Environmental modification, pacing, graded exposure, accommodation	Sensory / environmental	6, 7
Detoxification concerns	Hepatic, lymphatic, elimination	Foundational support (hydration, fiber, movement, sleep); **avoid aggressive protocols and speculative chelation**	Detox / hepatic	7

Environmental and accessibility accommodations. Sound: minimize background noise, avoid high-pitched tones and constant hums from electronics and HVAC where possible, offer quiet zones. Light: prefer natural and soft indirect lighting; reduce glare; avoid prolonged indoor tinted-lens use, which can worsen sensitivity through adaptation. Scent and air quality: minimize synthetic fragrance and chemical cleaning odors; ensure ventilation. Instruction format: offer visual, verbal, and kinesthetic options, and invite patients to indicate what works best for them today rather than assuming a fixed preference.

Appendix D: QIM Resource Guide

D.1 Referral Directory, Building a Brain-Injury Care Team

Framed by symptom and clinical question, matching Chapter 2's Assessment Pathways rather than a testing hierarchy. This is a true resource directory, not only a specialty-testing referral list.

Discipline	When to involve
Physiatrist / physical medicine and rehabilitation physician	Overall rehabilitation planning and coordination
Neurologist	Neurologic diagnosis, seizure risk, medication management
Neuropsychologist	Cognitive and psychological assessment, specialist-level diagnostics
Primary care clinician	Ongoing coordination, first point of contact for new symptoms
Cardiology or autonomic specialist	Suspected dysautonomia, orthostatic symptoms, palpitations
Sleep-medicine specialist	Persistent sleep disturbance, suspected sleep-disordered breathing
Vestibular physical therapist	Assessment-directed dizziness, balance, or gaze dysfunction
Physical therapist	General mobility, strength, and movement rehabilitation
Occupational therapist	Activities of daily living, cognitive-functional strategies
Speech-language pathologist	Communication, cognitive-linguistic function, swallowing
Audiologist	Hearing changes, tinnitus, auditory processing concerns
Rehabilitation optometrist	Vision therapy for convergence insufficiency, oculomotor dysfunction, visual-motion sensitivity
Neuro-ophthalmologist	Neurologic visual pathway conditions requiring medical/surgical ophthalmologic expertise, a different scope than rehabilitation optometry
Behavioral-health or trauma-informed mental-health professional	Mood, trauma history, engagement with care (*see Chapter 7*)
Registered dietitian nutritionist	Nutrition planning, medically supervised dietary changes
Gastroenterologist	GI symptoms, validated stool-marker interpretation

Discipline	When to involve
Endocrinologist	Suspected or established endocrine disorders, clinically indicated endocrine evaluation
Allergist/immunologist	Evaluation of suspected allergic or mast-cell disorders
Rheumatologist	Autoimmune/neuroimmune follow-up
Genetic counselor	Medically indicated genetic evaluation, family-history assessment, interpretation of clinically appropriate genetic testing, not every direct-to-consumer nutrigenomic panel
Clinical pharmacist	Medication interaction review, pharmacogenomic interpretation where clinically indicated
Medical toxicologist or physician with relevant training in occupational or environmental medicine	Environmental/heavy-metal exposure evaluation

D.2 Test Logistics, General Planning Ranges, Not Guarantees

Costs, turnaround times, availability, authorization requirements, and insurance coverage vary substantially by laboratory, geographic location, clinical indication, and payer. Verify current information before testing. Planning ranges below are general; individual timelines and coverage depend on your specific situation.

Clinical history and physical examination come first, before any of the testing below, they aren't a laboratory category, but the starting point every pathway in Chapter 2 builds from.

Test or assessment	Clinical question or purpose	Limitations and planning considerations	Typical specialist
Routine bloodwork (CBC, metabolic panel, thyroid, vitamin D, iron studies)	Broad first-line screening	Fastest turnaround; most consistently covered by insurance	Primary care clinician
MRI	Detailed structural evaluation, hemorrhage, contusion, diffuse axonal injury, atrophy, or alternative structural pathology	Longer turnaround; usually covered with referral	Neurologist, radiologist

Test or assessment	Clinical question or purpose	Limitations and planning considerations	Typical specialist
Brain-perfusion SPECT	Regional cerebral perfusion patterns; potentially complementary functional information when clinically indicated	Not specific to TBI; affected by technical and clinical variables; involves radiation exposure; should not independently determine diagnosis, prognosis, or treatment	Neurologist, physiatrist, nuclear-medicine physician, or appropriately qualified neuroimaging specialist

Test or assessment	Clinical question or purpose	Limitations and planning considerations	Typical specialist
Routine EEG	Seizures, epileptiform activity, and episodic changes in awareness when clinically suspected	A normal routine EEG does not exclude epilepsy; not a routine diagnostic test for persistent post-concussion symptoms	Neurologist, epileptologist, or clinical neurophysiologist
Prolonged, ambulatory, or video EEG	Infrequent or difficult-to-characterize events requiring longer observation and clinical correlation	Greater time, cost, and access burden; testing must match event frequency and clinical question	Neurologist or epileptologist

Test or assessment	Clinical question or purpose	Limitations and planning considerations	Typical specialist
Quantitative EEG (qEEG)	Computer-assisted analysis of EEG frequency, power, and related patterns	Findings are not specific to TBI; methods and clinical utility vary; should not independently determine diagnosis or treatment	Appropriately trained neurologist, clinical neurophysiologist, or qualified clinician working within scope
Neuropsychological testing	Cognitive and functional evaluation	Longer turnaround; usually covered with referral	Neuropsychologist
Validated stool/GI markers (e.g., inflammatory markers, pathogen panels)	Defined clinical questions about GI function	Moderate turnaround; coverage varies	An appropriately licensed healthcare professional with training relevant to the test, or a gastroenterologist

Test or assessment	Clinical question or purpose	Limitations and planning considerations	Typical specialist
Broad commercial microbiome profiling	Distinguished from validated GI markers above	Clinical actionability of broad profiling remains limited; results should be interpreted cautiously	An appropriately licensed healthcare professional with specific training in interpreting this category

Test or assessment	Clinical question or purpose	Limitations and planning considerations	Typical specialist
Organic acids testing	Varies by proposed use	Clinical validity and actionability vary considerably by the specific proposed use, interpretation complexity alone isn't the central limitation, and some applications lack established clinical utility	An appropriately licensed healthcare professional with training relevant to this specific test
Environmental/toxicant testing	Exposure-related evaluation	Coverage rarely extends here; requires exposure history to interpret meaningfully	Physician with relevant training in occupational or environmental medicine

Test or assessment	Clinical question or purpose	Limitations and planning considerations	Typical specialist
Genetic/genomic testing	Medically indicated genetic questions	Coverage varies by indication	Genetic counselor, clinical pharmacist, or ordering physician

Peripheral or urinary neurotransmitter panels are not a reliable measure of neurotransmitter activity in the brain and are not included in this table as a routine testing category.

No single imaging or electrophysiology test captures the entire brain, MRI examines structure, SPECT examines regional blood flow, and EEG records electrical activity. These are complementary, not interchangeable, and each should be selected to answer a defined clinical question (see Chapter 2 §2.3).

D.3 Biofeedback and Neurofeedback, Intervention, Not Diagnosis

Biofeedback is an intervention and self-regulation tool, not a diagnostic test, assessment shows a pattern, biofeedback helps a person practice changing one, and the two shouldn't be presented as the same category of thing.

Modality	Primary purpose	Considerations
HRV or respiratory biofeedback	Support awareness of breathing and cardiovascular regulation patterns (*see Chapter 4*)	Adjunctive tool; interpretation and tolerance vary; not diagnostic of dysautonomia
EMG biofeedback	Increase awareness of muscle activation and support tension or motor retraining goals	Placement and protocol should match the clinical question
Thermal biofeedback	Build awareness of peripheral temperature changes associated with arousal or circulation	Nonspecific signal; should not be interpreted as a diagnosis

Modality	Primary purpose	Considerations
EEG neurofeedback	Provide feedback from selected EEG features during a structured learning process	Evidence and protocols vary; requires careful artifact control and appropriately trained oversight; a diagnostic qEEG finding should not be assumed to automatically identify the correct neurofeedback protocol

Biofeedback should be selected according to the person's symptoms, goals, tolerance, cognitive capacity, and ability to interpret feedback without becoming overwhelmed or excessively focused on physiologic data, more information is not automatically more regulating. It can make an invisible physiologic process more visible, but shouldn't be presented as proving the cause of symptoms or as a substitute for comprehensive rehabilitation.

D.4 Before Ordering Any Test, Preanalytic Factors Checklist

- Fasting status and time since last meal
- Time of day (cortisol, testosterone, and other diurnal hormones)
- Menstrual cycle phase for sex-hormone testing
- Recent exercise (transiently affects inflammatory/metabolic markers)
- Recent or current infection/illness
- Current medications/supplements, and recent steroid use (e.g., biotin interference with immunoassays)
- Acute changes in medications
- Hydration status
- Specimen handling and transport time (organic acids, some hormones)
- Preparation requirements and appropriate waiting periods are test-specific, confirm with the ordering clinician and laboratory rather than relying on general guidance; this applies especially to antibiotic-use windows for stool/microbiome testing
- Whether any supplement should be withheld before testing, only under clinician or laboratory guidance, not on a general assumption

> A test can be analytically accurate and still clinically misleading if collection or interpretation is poor.

D.5 How to Evaluate a Device or Tool, Brand-Neutral Criteria

Whatever the device, a vagus nerve stimulator, an HRV biofeedback platform, a sensory-environment tool, the same questions apply before adopting it:

- **What is the mechanism, specifically?** Electrical stimulation and vibrotactile input are different mechanisms that produce different effects, even when marketed toward the same outcome. Don't assume interchangeability across mechanism types.
- **What evidence exists for the general modality versus this specific product?** A well-studied modality doesn't automatically transfer its evidence to every product using that mechanism.
- **Is there independent replication, or only manufacturer-funded research?**
- **Is the product a regulated medical device or a general-wellness product, and does its regulatory status apply to the exact intended use?** FDA clearance for one indication doesn't validate a different marketed use.
- **What are the contraindications for this specific device category?** Contraindications vary by device, the examples given anywhere in this book are screening prompts, not a universal or exhaustive list.
- **What does the device cost over the realistic period of use**, including subscriptions, consumables, and replacement parts?
- **For app-connected devices: what happens to the data?** Ask about data privacy, storage, and whether the data is shared with third parties.
- **Does the device require clinician oversight**, and is that oversight available?
- **What's the return policy**, and are there ongoing subscription costs beyond the initial purchase?
- **Is the device accessible** for the specific sensory, cognitive, motor, or visual limitations the patient has?
- **Would a simpler, lower-cost, or already-in-use tool answer the same clinical question first?**

D.6 Supplement and Nutraceutical Quality, Brand-Neutral Standards

- **Third-party verification.** Independent testing programs can provide information about identity, purity, contaminants, or label accuracy, depending on the specific program, this does not, by itself, demonstrate that a supplement is clinically effective.

- **Standardization.** A standardized percentage of the active compound improves product consistency, which can support plausibility, but standardization alone doesn't establish clinical benefit or safety.
- **Bioavailability and formulation.** Bioavailability claims should be supported by appropriate evidence, not marketing language, as Chapter 3 and Chapter 6 note for curcumin and CoQ10 specifically, the raw compound and the clinically effective delivery form aren't always the same thing.
- **Dose transparency.** The label should state the actual dose of active compound per serving. Proprietary blends limit dose transparency and make it difficult to know what's actually being taken.
- **Manufacturing standards.** Products manufactured in compliance with applicable current Good Manufacturing Practice (cGMP) requirements meet a baseline manufacturing standard, this is not proof of efficacy or independent content verification.
- **Additional label information worth checking:** lot number, expiration date, allergen disclosure, storage requirements, and adverse-event contact information.
- **A caution sign:** products making disease-treatment claims on their labeling are a red flag, regardless of other quality indicators.

D.7 Choosing a Qualified Practitioner for Specialized Testing

- Ask what specific clinical question a proposed test is meant to answer, and what would change about care based on an abnormal versus normal result, if nothing would change, that's a sign the test may not be necessary.
- Ask what the practitioner's specific licensure and training are relevant to the test being ordered, "an appropriately licensed healthcare professional with training relevant to the test and the patient's clinical needs" is a more accurate ask than assuming any one credential standardly covers this.
- Ask what the practitioner would do differently based on a positive versus negative result, before agreeing to the test.
- Ask about cost transparency up front, including what insurance is unlikely to cover.
- A practitioner who can explain *why* a test matters for your specific presentation, not just recite what it measures in general, is a good sign of genuine clinical reasoning.

D.8 Questions to Bring to Your Healthcare Team

- "What is this test/treatment meant to tell us, and what would change about my care based on the result?"
- "What's the evidence for this specifically, versus the general category it belongs to?"
- "What are the limitations of this test or treatment?"
- "Could this result be incidental, uncertain, or difficult to act upon?"
- "Could any medication or supplement I already use affect the result or create an interaction?"
- "What would you expect to see if this is working, and by when?"
- "How will we decide when to continue, modify, or stop?"
- "Who will coordinate these recommendations with the rest of my healthcare team?"
- "Is there a lower-cost or lower-risk option that would answer the same question first?"

D.9 Using This Guide Safely

This guide is designed to support informed conversations with your healthcare team, it is not a tool for self-diagnosis or self-treatment. New or worsening neurologic symptoms, seizures, repeated vomiting, worsening severe headache, double vision, slurred speech, marked confusion or behavioral change, or declining alertness require prompt medical assessment, not a self-directed testing or supplement decision. Testing, devices, and supplements should be individualized to your specific situation and reviewed with a qualified clinician rather than applied generally based on a symptom category.

This appendix reflects information available at the time of publication; evidence, regulatory status, costs, and insurance coverage evolve over time. Verify current status before acting on anything here rather than treating this guide as a permanent reference.

Appendix E: Sample Clinical Protocols

For insight, not prescription.

The following examples illustrate how core interventions may be adapted in QIM for ABI. **These are not universal protocols. They are starting points for clinical consideration.** Always assess individual readiness, therapeutic response, and scope of practice before applying any intervention, and adjust to the person rather than to the number.

> **A note on the ranges below.** Where the original manuscript gave specific dose and frequency ranges, those have been retained where they reflect ranges actually reported in clinical literature, and framed explicitly as starting points requiring individualization. They are not validated ABI protocols, and the evidence base does not support presenting them as such. Nothing here substitutes for clinical judgment, interaction checking, or coordination with prescribing clinicians.

Neurofeedback

Commonly delivered two to three times weekly in sessions of roughly 30 to 45 minutes, with courses often running 20 to 40 sessions and individualized to assessment findings. Regular clinician monitoring supports safe and adaptive use. Remember that qEEG findings alone do not prescribe a protocol, and that response should guide adjustment.

Nutritional Supplementation

Practitioners may explore mitochondrial support nutrients, with CoQ10 commonly used in the range of roughly 100 to 300 mg daily and NAD+ precursors in the range of roughly 250 to 500 mg daily, adjusted to symptom burden and tolerance. Periodic reassessment is sensible where testing is being used. **Check interactions, particularly with anticoagulants and other prescribed medications, and consider cost as a clinical variable.** Evidence for these in ABI specifically is mechanistic rather than outcome-based.

Gut-Brain Support

Probiotics, glutamine (commonly around 5 to 10 g daily), or anti-inflammatory nutrition may be introduced to support gut integrity and vagal signaling. **Start low and progress slowly**, since many patients in this population require gradual onboarding to avoid GI discomfort. Probiotic selection should be strain-appropriate to the indication rather than chosen by CFU count alone. Screen for red-flag GI symptoms before managing digestive complaints integratively.

Mindfulness and Meditation

Short sessions of roughly 5 to 10 minutes support emotional regulation, interoceptive awareness, and cognitive clarity, and are more sustainable than longer sessions early on. Patients with ABI often benefit from guided or sensory-rich forms that do not demand sustained unsupported attention. **Screen for trauma activation**: mind-body practices can surface unresolved trauma, so ensure grounding tools, consent, and referral pathways are in place.

Dual-Task Cognitive Exercises

These target cross-domain activation, for example walking while problem-solving, or balancing while generating category items. Sessions may begin around 10 to 15 minutes and increase in complexity over time. **Scale to attention span, fatigue, and physical safety**, and stop before the point of crash rather than after it.

PEMF Therapy

Included for reference. PEMF requires specialized equipment and training. Frequencies in the low-hertz range are commonly discussed in the literature, but device parameters vary widely and **there is no established universal protocol for ABI**. Begin at the lowest intensity, increase gradually, and monitor for overstimulation and rebound fatigue, which are common in this population.

A Sample "Day in the Life"

The original manuscript promised a structured daily routine as a tangible example of integrative ABI care. A workable shape, to be adapted rather than followed:

- **Morning.** Consistent wake time. Natural light exposure within the first hour, outdoors where possible. Hydration with attention to electrolytes. Protein-containing breakfast. A brief regulation practice, breathwork or short mindfulness, before the day's demands begin.
- **Midday.** The most cognitively demanding work scheduled when energy is typically best. Structured pacing with deliberate rest before fatigue, not after. Movement appropriate to tolerance.

- **Afternoon.** Therapy or active rehabilitation work if scheduled, with regulation built into the session rather than added at the end. Attention to blood sugar stability across the afternoon.
- **Evening.** Reduced light and screen exposure. A wind-down routine that consistently signals downshift. Warm bath, magnesium, calming herbal tea, or gentle stretching as suits the person. Consistent sleep timing.

The shape matters more than the specifics: anchor the day with light and consistent timing, front-load demand, build in rest before crash, and give the nervous system a reliable signal that the day is ending.

References

Every work cited in this guide appears below. Sources are grouped alphabetically.

Breit, S., Kupferberg, A., Rogler, G., & Hasler, G. (2018). Vagus nerve as modulator of the brain-gut axis in psychiatric and inflammatory disorders. Frontiers in Psychiatry, 9, 44.

Buccino, G. (2014). Action observation treatment: A novel tool in neurorehabilitation. Philosophical Transactions of the Royal Society B: Biological Sciences, 369(1644), 20130185. https://doi.org/10.1098/rstb.2013.0185 (PMID 24778380)

Carabotti, M., Scirocco, A., Maselli, M. A., & Severi, C. (2015). The gut-brain axis: Interactions between enteric microbiota, central and enteric nervous systems. Annals of Gastroenterology, 28(2), 203-209. (PMID 25830558)

Cicerone, K. D., Goldin, Y., Ganci, K., Rosenbaum, A., Wethe, J. V., Langenbahn, D. M., Malec, J. F., Bergquist, T. F., Kingsley, K., Nagele, D., Trexler, L., Fraas, M., Bogdanova, Y., & Harley, J. P. (2019). Evidence-based cognitive rehabilitation: Systematic review of the literature from 2009 through 2014. Archives of Physical Medicine and Rehabilitation, 100(8), 1515-1533. https://doi.org/10.1016/j.apmr.2019.02.011 (PMID 30926291)

Cryan, J. F., O'Riordan, K. J., Cowan, C. S. M., Sandhu, K. V., Bastiaanssen, T. F. S., Boehme, M., ... & Dinan, T. G. (2019). The microbiota-gut-brain axis. Physiological Reviews, 99(4), 1877-2013.

Edinger, J. D., & Carney, C. E. (2015). Overcoming insomnia: A cognitive-behavioral therapy approach. Oxford University Press.

Franceschini, M., Agosti, M., Cantagallo, A., Sale, P., Mancuso, M., & Buccino, G. (2010). Mirror neurons: Action observation treatment as a tool in stroke rehabilitation. European Journal of Physical and Rehabilitation Medicine, 46(4), 517-523.

Galeno, E., Pullano, E., Mourad, F., Galeoto, G., & Frontani, F. (2022). Effectiveness of vestibular rehabilitation after concussion: A systematic review of randomised controlled trials. Healthcare, 11(1), 90. https://doi.org/10.3390/healthcare11010090

Garrison, K. A., Winstein, C. J., & Aziz-Zadeh, L. (2010). The mirror neuron system: A neural substrate for methods in stroke rehabilitation. Neurorehabilitation and Neural Repair, 24(5), 404-412. https://doi.org/10.1177/1545968309354536

Giza, C. C., & Hovda, D. A. (2014). The new neurometabolic cascade of concussion. Neurosurgery, 75(Supplement_4), S24-S33.

Gruzelier, J. H. (2014). EEG-neurofeedback for optimising performance. I: A review of cognitive and affective outcome in healthy participants. Neuroscience & Biobehavioral Reviews, 44, 124-141.

Hall, E. D., Wang, J. A., Bosken, J. M., & Singh, I. N. (2010). Lipid peroxidation in brain or spinal cord mitochondria after injury. Journal of Bioenergetics and Biomembranes, 42(6), 431-434.

Hiebert, J. B., Shen, Q., Thimmesch, A. R., & Pierce, J. D. (2015). Traumatic brain injury and mitochondrial dysfunction. The American Journal of the Medical Sciences, 350(2), 132-138. https://doi.org/10.1097/MAJ.0000000000000506 (PMID 26083647)

Hsieh, Y. W., Lin, Y. H., Zhu, J. D., Wu, C. Y., Lin, Y. P., & Chen, C. C. (2020). Treatment effects of upper limb action observation therapy and mirror therapy on rehabilitation outcomes after subacute stroke: A pilot study. Behavioural Neurology, 2020, 6250524. https://doi.org/10.1155/2020/6250524 (PMID 32377266)

Jackson, P. L., Lafleur, M. F., Malouin, F., Richards, C. L., & Doyon, J. (2001). Potential role of mental practice using motor imagery in neurologic rehabilitation. Archives of Physical Medicine and Rehabilitation, 82(8), 1133-1141.

Jerath, R., Edry, J. W., Barnes, V. A., & Jerath, V. (2006). Physiology of long pranayamic breathing: Neural, respiratory, and cardiovascular correlates. Medical Hypotheses, 67(3), 566-571.

Kennedy, M. R. T., et al. (2008). Intervention for executive functions after traumatic brain injury: A systematic review, meta-analysis, and clinical recommendations. Neuropsychological Rehabilitation, 18(3), 257-299.

Kleim, J. A., & Jones, T. A. (2008). Principles of experience-dependent neural plasticity: Implications for rehabilitation after brain damage. Journal of Speech, Language, and Hearing Research, 51(1), S225-S239.

Kolb, B., & Gibb, R. (2011). Brain plasticity and behaviour in the developing brain. Journal of the Canadian Academy of Child and Adolescent Psychiatry, 20(4), 265-276.

Loane, D. J., & Kumar, A. (2016). Microglia in the TBI brain: The good, the bad, and the dysregulated. Experimental Neurology, 275(Pt 3), 316-327.

Lu, H. C., Gevirtz, R., Yang, C. C., & Hauson, A. O. (2023). Heart rate variability biofeedback for mild traumatic brain injury: A randomized-controlled study. Applied Psychophysiology and Biofeedback, 48(4), 405-421. https://doi.org/10.1007/s10484-023-09592-4

Ly, C., Greb, A. C., Cameron, L. P., Wong, J. M., Barragan, E. V., Wilson, P. C., ... Olson, D. E. (2018). Psychedelics promote structural and functional neural plasticity. Cell Reports, 23(11), 3170-3182. https://doi.org/10.1016/j.celrep.2018.05.022 (PMID 29898390)

Mercier, L. J., Batycky, J., Campbell, C., Schneider, K., Smirl, J., & Debert, C. T. (2022). Autonomic dysfunction in adults following mild traumatic brain injury: A systematic review. NeuroRehabilitation, 50(1), 3-32. https://doi.org/10.3233/NRE-210243

Naeser, M. A., Saltmarche, A., Krengel, M. H., Hamblin, M. R., & Knight, J. A. (2011). Improved cognitive function after transcranial, light-emitting diode treatments in chronic, traumatic brain injury: Two case reports. Photomedicine and Laser Surgery, 29(5), 351-358. https://doi.org/10.1089/pho.2010.2814 (PMID 21182447)

Pathare, N., Sushilkumar, S., Haley, L., Jain, S., & Osier, N. N. (2020). The impact of traumatic brain injury on microbiome composition: A systematic review. Biological Research for Nursing, 22(4), 495-505. https://doi.org/10.1177/1099800420943961 (PMID 32720519)

Prins, M. L., & Matsumoto, J. H. (2014). The collective therapeutic potential of cerebral ketone metabolism in traumatic brain injury. Journal of Lipid Research, 55(12), 2450-2457. https://doi.org/10.1194/jlr.R046706

Rizzolatti, G., & Craighero, L. (2004). The mirror-neuron system. Annual Review of Neuroscience, 27, 169-192.

Rytter, H. M., Graff, H. J., Henriksen, H. K., Aaen, N., Hartvigsen, J., Hoegh, M., Nisted, I., Naess-Schmidt, E. T., Pedersen, L. L., Schytz, H. W., Thastum, M. M., Zerlang, B., & Callesen, H. E. (2021). Nonpharmacological treatment of persistent postconcussion symptoms in adults: A systematic review and meta-analysis and guideline recommendation. JAMA Network Open, 4(11), e2132221. https://doi.org/10.1001/jamanetworkopen.2021.32221 (PMID 34751759)

Slutsky, I., et al. (2010). Basal GABA regulates GABA(B) receptor conformation and release probability at single hippocampal synapses. Neuron, 67(2), 253-267.

Substance Abuse and Mental Health Services Administration. (2014). SAMHSA's concept of trauma and guidance for a trauma-informed approach (HHS Publication No. SMA 14-4884). Rockville, MD: Substance Abuse and Mental Health Services Administration.

Tan, C. L., Alavi, S. A., Baldeweg, S. E., Belli, A., Carson, A., Feeney, C., Goldstone, A. P., Greenwood, R., Menon, D. K., Simpson, H. L., Toogood, A. A., Gurnell, M., & Hutchinson, P. J. (2017). The screening and management of pituitary dysfunction following traumatic brain injury in adults: British Neurotrauma Group guidance. Journal of Neurology, Neurosurgery & Psychiatry, 88(11), 971-981. https://doi.org/10.1136/jnnp-2016-315500 (PMID 28860331)

Tang, Y. Y., Ma, Y., Wang, J., Fan, Y., Feng, S., Lu, Q., ... & Posner, M. I. (2007). Short-term meditation training improves attention and self-regulation. Proceedings of the National Academy of Sciences, 104(43), 17152-17156.

Thibault, R. T., Lifshitz, M., & Raz, A. (2016). The self-regulating brain and neurofeedback: Experimental science and clinical promise. Cortex, 74, 247-261. https://doi.org/10.1016/j.cortex.2015.10.024 (PMID 26706052)

Zafonte, R. D., Bagiella, E., Ansel, B. M., Novack, T. A., Friedewald, W. T., Hesdorffer, D. C., ... Dikmen, S. S. (2012). Effect of citicoline on functional and cognitive status among patients with traumatic brain injury: Citicoline Brain Injury Treatment Trial (COBRIT). JAMA, 308(19), 1993-2000. https://doi.org/10.1001/jama.2012.13256 (PMID 23168823)

Zhang, Z., Wang, Y., & Xiang, J. (2022). Neuroprotective effects of magnesium and curcumin in acquired brain injury. Molecular Neurobiology, 59(3), 1504-1521.

About the Author

Dr. Sarah Young, IMD, PhD, CCC-SLP, is a board-certified Doctor of Integrative Medicine, medical speech-language pathologist, and founder of the NeuroSynergy Health Institute. With over a decade of experience in neurorehabilitation, Dr. Young blends neuroscience, functional medicine, and holistic healing to help individuals recover from acquired brain injury (ABI), trauma, and chronic illness.

After navigating multiple brain injuries herself, Dr. Young became a fierce advocate for patient-centered care, neuroplasticity-driven healing, and quantum integrative medicine. Her work bridges science and soul, bringing together evidence-informed protocols, energy-based tools, and compassionate connection.

When she is not writing or teaching, she supports clients through personalized recovery programs and community healing workshops. Her mission is simple: to restore clarity, vitality, and wholeness, one brain and body at a time.

Learn more at www.NeuroSynergyHealth.com

Stay Connected. Follow Dr. Sarah and NeuroSynergy Health Institute for tools, tips, and encouragement on the healing journey:

- Website: www.NeuroSynergyHealth.com
- Instagram: @NeuroSynergyHealth
- Facebook: @NeuroSynergyHealth
- YouTube: @neurosynergyhealth
- Email: drsarahyoung@NeuroSynergyHealth.com

www.ingramcontent.com/pod-product-compliance
Lightning Source LLC
LaVergne TN
LVHW060038210926
848481LV00013B/3893